Palgrave Macmillan Studies in Family and Intimate Life
Series Standing Order ISBN 978–0–230–51748–6 Hardback
                              978–0–230–24924–0 Paperback
(*outside North America only*)

You can receive future titles in this series as they are published by placing a standing order. Please contact your bookseller or, in case of difficulty, write to us at the address below with your name and address, the title of the series and the ISBN quoted above.

Customer Services Department, Macmillan Distribution Ltd, Houndmills, Basingstoke, Hampshire RG21 6XS, England

Displaying Families

A New Concept for the Sociology of Family Life

Edited By
Esther Dermott
University of Bristol, UK

and

Julie Seymour
University of Hull, UK

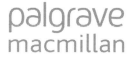

Selection and editorial matter © Esther Dermott and Julie Seymour 2011
Individual chapters © their respective authors 2011

All rights reserved. No reproduction, copy or transmission of this
publication may be made without written permission.

No portion of this publication may be reproduced, copied or transmitted
save with written permission or in accordance with the provisions of the
Copyright, Designs and Patents Act 1988, or under the terms of any licence
permitting limited copying issued by the Copyright Licensing Agency,
Saffron House, 6–10 Kirby Street, London EC1N 8TS.

Any person who does any unauthorized act in relation to this publication
may be liable to criminal prosecution and civil claims for damages.

The authors have asserted their rights to be identified as the authors of this
work in accordance with the Copyright, Designs and Patents Act 1988.

First published 2011 by
PALGRAVE MACMILLAN

Palgrave Macmillan in the UK is an imprint of Macmillan Publishers Limited,
registered in England, company number 785998, of Houndmills, Basingstoke,
Hampshire RG21 6XS.

Palgrave Macmillan in the US is a division of St Martin's Press LLC,
175 Fifth Avenue, New York, NY 10010.

Palgrave Macmillan is the global academic imprint of the above companies
and has companies and representatives throughout the world.

Palgrave® and Macmillan® are registered trademarks in the United States,
the United Kingdom, Europe and other countries

ISBN: 978–0–230–24613–3 hardback

This book is printed on paper suitable for recycling and made from fully
managed and sustained forest sources. Logging, pulping and manufacturing
processes are expected to conform to the environmental regulations of the
country of origin.

A catalogue record for this book is available from the British Library.

Library of Congress Cataloging-in-Publication Data

Displaying families : a new concept for the sociology of family life /
edited by Julie Seymour, Esther Dermott.
    p. cm.—(Palgrave Macmillan studies in family and intimate life)
Includes bibliographical references and index.
ISBN 978–0–230–24613–3 (alk. paper)
1. Families. I. Seymour, Julie. II. Dermott, Esther, 1973–

HQ519.D57 2011
306.850941—dc22   2011013818

10 9 8 7 6 5 4 3 2 1
20 19 18 17 16 15 14 13 12 11

Printed and bound in the United States of America

Contents

Acknowledgements

We are grateful to the British Sociological Association for their assistance in organising the original day seminar which led to this volume and to Clare Whitfield for her smooth administration during the event. We would like to thank the members of the BSA Family Study Group who contributed to what was an energising and thought-provoking day and for those whose enthusiasm has sustained the project during its gestation. Our thanks also go to David Morgan, Lynn Jamieson and Graham Allan, the editors of the *Studies in Family and Intimate Life* series and Philippa Grand and Olivia Middleton at Palgrave Macmillan for their support and helpfulness.

Kathy Almack's chapter first appeared in a slightly different form as Almack, K. (2008) 'Display Work: Lesbian Parent Couples and their Families of Origin Negotiating New Kin Relationships', *Sociology*, 42, 1183–99, Sage.

Notes on Contributors

Kathryn Almack is Senior Research Fellow in Palliative and End of Life Studies at the University of Nottingham. Her research is underpinned by sociological research interests, particularly concerning the dynamics and diversity of family lives and research in sensitive and ethically challenging areas such as palliative and end of life studies. Recent publications include concerns about end of life care and on bereavement for lesbian, gay and bisexual older people (2010) and lesbian parent couples (2008).

Esther Dermott is Senior Lecturer in Sociology at the University of Bristol, U.K. She is the author of *Intimate Fatherhood* (Routledge, 2008) and has written widely on fathering, intimacy and work. She is currently writing a new book, *Intimacy and Personal Life* for Palgrave and is working on the gender and parenting elements of a major ESRC-funded project on poverty and social exclusion in the U.K.

Nika Dorrer works part-time as Researcher at Glasgow Caledonian University, Scotland, while she completes her postgraduate training as social worker. She has been involved in research on the interrelation between social contexts, identity and well-being with a particular focus on young people and has conducted studies in Tobago and Scotland, in schools, and in voluntary and statutory care settings.

Andrea Doucet is Professor of Sociology at Carleton University in Ottawa, Canada. She is the author of *Do Men Mother?* (2006), which received the John Porter Tradition of Excellence Book Award from the Canadian Sociology Association, and co-author of *Gender Relations: Intersectionality and Beyond* (2008) and the forthcoming *A Guide through Qualitative Analysis: Listening, Seeing and Reading Narrative Data*. She has published widely on themes of gender, work and care; mothering and fathering; care and justice; reflexive sociology; and knowledge construction processes. She is the Editor of the journal *Fathering* and is currently completing a book on North American primary breadwinning mothers.

Ruth Emond is a part-time Senior Lecturer in the Department of Applied Social Science at the University of Stirling. She teaches on the social work programme and has undertaken research with children in public care in the U.K., Ireland and Cambodia. She is particularly interested in children's friendships and social networks and how these affect their experiences of being 'looked after'. The other half of the week she works as a play therapist and social worker at the Family Change Project in Perth. Here she works with children and young people who have experienced trauma.

Janet Finch is Honorary Professor of Sociology at Manchester University, where she is a member of the Morgan Centre for the Study of Relationships and Personal Life. Until 2010 she was Vice Chancellor of Keele University, a position which she had held for 15 years. Her research interests in the sociology of family relationships have focused mainly on relationships across generations in kin networks. She is the author of the article on 'Displaying Families' in *Sociology* (2007), which provided the stimulus for this book.

Jacqui Gabb of the Department of Social Policy and Criminology at The Open University has developed inter-disciplinary qualitative mixed methods approaches for the study of family relationships. She is author of *Researching Intimacy in Families* (2008) which won the 2009 BSA Philip Abrams Memorial Prize. She has particular interests in the areas of families, personal relationships, intimacy, emotions, sexuality and gender. She is co-convenor of the BSA Families and Relationships Study Group and Chair of the Editorial Board for *Sociological Research Online.*

Jo Haynes is Lecturer in Sociology at the University of Bristol. She has conducted extensive research on ethnicity/race and music/culture, including a qualitative study of the British world music scene. Her main research interests are focused on issues of racialisation within music and other settings such as the family and education. Her previous work includes governmental research dedicated to the experiences of African Caribbean pupils in education and research on film audiences and censorship.

Brian Heaphy is Senior Lecturer in Sociology at the University of Manchester. He has researched the implications of social change for relational life through studies of sexualities, families and intimacies, ageing and living with HIV. He is currently researching young couples' Civil Partnerships. His publications include the books *Same Sex Intimacies* (Routledge, 2001, with Jeffery Weeks and Catherine Donovan) and *Late Modernity and Social Change* (Routledge).

Kahryn Hughes is in the School of Sociology and Social Policy at the University of Leeds and researches individuals and groups traditionally considered hard-to-reach by the academic community. She is interested in understanding inter-generational poverty within families and across localities, relational processes of identity constitution and maintenance and theorising social networks in the context of low-income communities. This contribution draws from *New Forms of Participation: Internet Gambling and the Role of the Family*, funded under the ESRC/RIGT initiative.

Mary Jane Kehily is Senior Lecturer in Childhood and Youth Studies at the Open University, U.K. She has research interests in gender and sexuality, narrative and identity and popular culture and has published widely on these themes. Her books include: *Gender, Sexuality and Schooling, Shifting Agendas in Social Learning,* (Routledge, 2002), *An Introduction to Childhood Studies* (Open University Press/McGraw Hill, 2008), *Understanding Youth, Perspectives, Identities and Practices* (London: Sage/The Open University, 2007) and, with Anoop Nayak, *Gender, Youth and Culture, Young Masculinities and Femininities* (Palgrave, 2008).

Ian McIntosh is Senior Lecturer in Sociology in the Department of Applied Social Science, University of Stirling, Scotland, U.K. He was recently involved in an ESRC-funded project which investigated the role of food within residential homes for young people and is the co-author of *English People in Scotland: An Invisible Minority* (2008).

Samantha Punch is Senior Lecturer in Sociology in the Department of Applied Social Science at the University of Stirling in Scotland. Her research interests are located within the sociology of childhood (including sibling relationships and birth order, food practices in residential care, rural childhoods in Bolivia) and the sociology of development (including household livelihoods in Asia and Latin America, migration and child labour).

Roísín Ryan-Flood is Senior Lecturer in Sociology and Director of the Centre for Intimate and Sexual Citizenship (CISC) at the

University of Essex. Her research interests include gender, sexuality, citizenship, kinship and migration. She also has a long-standing interest in feminist epistemology and methodology. Her publications include the monograph *Lesbian Motherhood: Gender, Families and Sexual Citizenship* (Palgrave, 2009) and a co-edited book (with Rosalind Gill), *Silence and Secrecy in the Research Process: Feminist Reflections* (Routledge, 2009). Her current research explores sexual citizenship and diaspora.

Julie Seymour is Senior Lecturer in Social Research in the Department of Social Sciences at the University of Hull. She has written about the allocation of, and negotiations around, the divisions of resources in the family in relation to domestic labour, disability and informal caring, space, emotional labour and time. Recent publications include contributions to *Geographies of Children, Youth and Families* (Routledge, 2011) and *Listening to the Children* (Berghahn, 2011). She is currently writing a book on *Family Practices and Spatiality*.

Liz Short is Researcher at the School of Social Sciences and Psychology at Victoria University, Australia, where she also teaches community and clinical psychology. She has worked extensively in the areas of community and clinical psychology (with a specialisation in child, adolescent and family psychology), including research, policy and service system analysis and development, community development and health promotion. Her research and writing focuses mainly on diverse families, lesbian-parented families, motherhood, gender, violence against women, and the socio-political determinants of health and well-being.

Rachel Thomson is Professor of Social Research in the Faculty of Health and Social Care at the Open University where she develops multi-media courses in the field of childhood, youth and personal life. She has research interests in transitions across the life course and in methodological strategies for describing and understanding the interplay of personal, social and historical change/continuity. Recent joint publications include *Inventing Adulthoods* (2007), *Unfolding Lives* (2009), *Researching Social Change* (2009) and *Making Modern Mothers* (2011).

Gill Valentine is Professor of Human Geography at the University of Leeds. Her research interests include social identities, citizenship and belonging; geographies of childhood, families and parenting; and consumption cultures. Gill's has (co)authored/edited 14 books and over one-hundred articles. Her books include *Public Space and the Culture of Childhood* (2004) and *CyberKids: Children and the Information Age* (2003).

Part I
Evaluating the Concept

1
Developing 'Displaying Families': A Possibility for the Future of the Sociology of Personal Life

Esther Dermott and Julie Seymour

Definition and origins

When Finch introduced the idea of 'displaying family' her principal aim was to start a discussion and encourage others 'to refine the concept as well as to use it' (2007: 65). We feel that this volume takes up this challenge and, in doing so, offers a discussion of emerging intellectual debates in family sociology along with contemporary accounts of meaningful family practices. As such it reflects the need for 'grounded, contextualised studies of family and intimacy' which also highlight the possibility of 'alternative, yet to be explored dimensions to the way people connect with one another' (Gillies 2003: 19).

The reason for our decision to compile an edited collection on 'Displaying Families' was because we felt that this concept did two things: it reflected important developments in contemporary thinking about family life and provided a useful additional tool for sociologists engaged in conducting research in this area. In this introductory chapter, we explain the origins of the volume and make the case as to why we believe it can provide a significant contribution to the field. We have avoided simply outlining the content of subsequent chapters in detail or second guessing how Janet Finch herself would respond to their content (indeed, this is unnecessary as she has generously contributed an afterword to the collection in which she comments on how the contributions presented here have used, developed and critiqued her concept; see Chapter 11). Instead, in arguing for the usefulness of 'displaying families', we draw attention to two significant issues we believe sociologists working in the area of 'family' need to address and to which 'displaying families' can make a contribution, those of individualisation and diversity. We then discuss two more particular concerns (audience and personal relationships) which we feel the concept of display illuminates and speaks to directly. We therefore focus mainly on the context for the addition of this new concept and how it can move thinking in the field forward.

The concept of 'displaying families' was initially outlined by the eminent family sociologist Professor Dame Janet Finch in 2007 in an article published in *Sociology*. Without wishing to restate her entire argument in detail here, it is worthwhile to offer a brief précis for those not acquainted with the concept. She explicitly links 'displaying families' to David Morgan's (1996) influential idea of family practices in which the activities of families – the doing of family life – are prioritised as a research focus over the construction of what a family is – who 'counts' as family. However, she goes further and argues that this idea needs to be expanded because *'families need to be "displayed" as well as "done"'* (Finch 2007: 66, original emphasis). She defines 'display' as 'the process by which individuals, and groups of individuals, convey to each other and to relevant audiences that certain of their actions do constitute 'doing family things' and thereby confirm that these relationships are 'family' relationships' (Finch 2007: 67). By suggesting this addition to the 'sociological tool kit' (Finch 2007: 65), she seeks to 'emphasize the fundamentally social nature of family practices' (Finch 2007: 67). In her development of the concept she addresses three elements: *'why* is display important in contemporary families; *how* is displaying done; *to whom* do "my family relationships" need to be displayed?' (Finch 2007: 67, original emphasis).

In conversations with colleagues we became aware that a number of people were immediately engaging with the concept, debating its value and applying it to their own empirical research. Since the idea had stimulated so much interest we decided to harness this enthusiasm and, under the auspices of the British Sociological Association's Family Study Group, organised a one-day seminar which would allow academics to present contributions exploring the idea based on their own ongoing or recently completed research and to engage in academic dialogue around how the original concept could or should be modified. Professor Finch argued that her intention was for 'display' to be understood in two senses: 'as an activity characteristic of contemporary families, and as an analytical concept' (2007: 78). It was partly this attribute of the concept – because the idea constituted both a theoretical intervention and a practical tool that could be 'worked with' – that we believed a wide range of academics working in the field of family research would be able to engage with it and find it useful. Finch also emphasised throughout the original article that the analysis she presented was 'provisional' and explicitly expressed the wish for other researchers to not only work with it, but also to hone and develop it. This expansive invitation meant that sociologists of family life had significant scope for exploring, interrogating and reconfiguring displaying families in a way that exposed a number of current concerns with how we examine and gain understanding about personal life today. Our feeling that the idea of 'displaying families' had merit and the potential for further development has since been confirmed by a small but growing body of published work associated with it (Almack 2008; James and Curtis 2010; Haldar and Waerdahl 2009).

Presenters at the seminar were, in particular, directed towards the questions raised at the end of Finch's article: is 'display' a useful addition to the repertoire of existing concepts which sociologists use to analyse families? What is the potential span of the concept? Is it possible to 'do' family without display? Additionally, as Finch herself states, the initial article focused to a greater degree on *why* display is important in contemporary families rather than on the *how* and *to whom* questions which she also posed. This left open the possibility that these latter questions could be given greater attention. The contributions and debate that resulted were stimulating and of a high quality – so much so that we felt the discussion should be reproduced and extended through an edited collection, allowing a wider audience to have access to the thinking about and around the concept. In our call for contributions to this collection, the same set of questions provided our starting point and we encouraged authors to take the opportunity to critically engage with the concept and suggest refinements, as well as adopting the concept for 'thinking with' in relation to their own research. All the published contributions responded to the request with enthusiasm and in selecting chapters for inclusion, we sought to reflect both the breadth of current sociological research concerned with 'family' and the variety of ways in which authors could 'take on' the idea of 'displaying families'. The result is that chapters in this collection examine the concept of 'displaying family' from a range of theoretical, empirical, epistemological and disciplinary viewpoints and from a variety of subject positions. The range of substantive themes covered at the initial seminar is reflected in the papers selected for this edited collection, including papers on lesbian parenting, internet gambling and experiences within a residential children's home. These have been supplemented by chapters on other areas of family that are of contemporary relevance: fathering, first time motherhood, raising families in the workplace, and mixed ethnicity. In considering the tools used to 'display families', our authors discuss variously the material objects, embodied actions, namings and narratives employed by those they researched. The book therefore engages with a broad range of concerns that are pertinent to studies of family and personal relationships, and reflects the richness of contemporary family studies: chapters address issues of sexuality, ethnicity, gender, space, work-life balance and consumption. Throughout the contributions, authors discuss how 'displaying family' can be examined using varied and, increasingly, innovative methodological techniques. The hope is that this volume, therefore, offers a new contribution to both theoretical and empirical understandings of family life.

Chapter outlines

The following two chapters in Part I, by Brian Heaphy and Jacqui Gabb, respectively, provide a robust evaluation and critique of the concept of displaying family; both offer warnings around what they consider to be possible problematic consequences of adopting the concept as well as discussing how it could be valuable. Heaphy makes suggestions as to how the concept could (and should) be refined in order that thinking on personal lives takes seriously 'the power and politics of contemporary relational life' (Chapter 2). Focussing on the 'family' aspect of displaying families, Heaphy argues that it is important that using this concept does not result in other relational displays being downgraded. Gabb argues that 'displaying families' is most useful if it is adopted as a 'sensitising concept' which alerts us to ways in which some family practices are considered 'troublesome' and, with similarities to Heaphy, warns against any tendency to prioritise only displays that are viewed as 'legitimate'. She also questions whether display is adequate as a tool for exploring the *interiority* of relationships.

The chapters in Part II use empirical studies of family life to engage with the concept of 'displaying families' and explore if and how it can be usefully applied in a range of different contexts. In doing so, they use 'displaying families' as a tool with which to think about their data in new ways but also use their empirical findings to shed evaluative light on particular aspects of the concept. Kehily and Thomson (Chapter 4) reflect on a particular moment in the lifecourse which is characterised by an intensification of display, namely conception and the public recognition of pregnancy. By examining how mothers-to-be embark on a 'maternal project that creates a "new" family' (Chapter 4), they suggest that there are a number of audiences to whom acts of display may be addressed and that displaying practices need to be recognised as existing within a broader landscape of cultural meaning. Andrea Doucet (Chapter 5) and Kathryn Almack (Chapter 6) also address the substantive topic of parenthood, each focusing on parenting 'whose contours are not easily recognised' (Almack: Chapter 6). Doucet focuses on fathers who are doing care differently by taking on the role of primary or shared caregivers, while Almack looks at lesbian parent families' relationships with their families of origin. Both, therefore, foreground the 'degrees of intensity' aspect of Finch's concept. Doucet argues that intensity of display is related to social and ideological changes more than individual circumstances. Further, her chapter highlights the way in which the actor who is 'displaying' and those who witness the displaying may interpret the practices in different ways, with fathers having to work hard to ensure that their displays of family are considered legitimate. Almack also raises the issue of legitimacy, noting that we need to be alert to displays which have not been successful and suggesting that engaging with the subject of the reception of display forces us to acknowledge that there are many layers to and different interpretations of a particular practice which is on display. Almack's chapter first appeared in a slightly different form in *Sociology* (2008) and this early application of the concept of displaying family has allowed us to invite two further scholars in the field of lesbian parenting (Short and Ryan-Flood) to discuss and comment on Almack's initial exploration.

In Chapter 7, Hughes and Valentine alert us to the way in which the negotiation of problematic internet gambling must be understood as existing within a set of 'threatened' family relations that must be worked on over time, and also highlight how the absence of appropriate displays of family need to be managed. The second issue – the presence or absence of display – chimes with the chapters of Doucet, Almack and Gabb who comment on the existence of non-displays and negative displays as well as those that 'work'. Haynes and Dermott (Chapter 8) consider how 'displaying family' can be usefully applied in relation to mixed ethnicity. They are concerned with who constitutes the audience for display and question the extent to which this audience can be chosen by those engaged in practices of display. They nevertheless embrace 'displaying family' as part of the shift towards a focus on practices which could manage to free studies of mixed ethnicity from overly prescribed categories. The chapters of Seymour (Chapter 9) and McIntosh and colleagues (Chapter 10) emphasise the importance of paying attention to the location in which displays of family take place. Looking at spaces which are not only private homes but merge domestic space, workplace and (for McIntosh et al.) institution, they both note how these sites (family-run hotels and children's care homes, respectively) require different kinds of display from actors and impose limitations on what can be displayed because of social restrictions on the kinds of social interaction considered appropriate.

Current issues and challenges for sociologists of family life

The last few years have seen a resurgence in sociological work around families. While popular interest in how we construct and manage our personal relationships has never really diminished, for a few decades those most engaged with describing and explaining contemporary families were located in other disciplines such as psychology or policy studies. Sociologists in turn became more excited by other areas of research and the sociology of family life became rather passé as a subject of study. (Of course much interesting research was still conducted but it lost any claim to being fashionable.) Happily, this is no longer the case and research within the sociology of family life (now often bracketed as part of a larger package along with intimacy and personal relationships) is flourishing once more.

Current theorising and empirical work have taken up the challenges posed by research in the last three decades. As Gillies (2003) describes, recent explorations of family life have been partly justified by convincing arguments that families remain of huge significance to individuals. At the same time, analyses have had to engage with discussions of the 1980s and 1990s which moved towards an emphasis on the lived experience of family and household members and its contingent and negotiated nature (Gillies 2003: 8–9). With this as the background for current sociological research on family we highlight in more detail here two ongoing, 'big' issues; those of individualisation and diversity. The first raises how, in the light of debates about individualisation and reflexivity, we find ways to integrate the ongoing significance of older social divisions with the acknowledged loosening of restrictions around what is acceptable in personal life. The second issue, relating to diversity and inter-sectionality, questions how to engage with debates and dilemmas which focus on particular types of family while also managing to develop deeper sociological understanding of families more generally. We suggest that 'displaying families' may be useful in dealing with both of these concerns because of its position within important frameworks for the analysis of families.

Challenging 'family': individualisation

Perhaps one reason why the sociology of families faded from view somewhat is that it took some time to deal with the individualisation thesis which gained currency in the 1990s. The theme of individualisation, promoted by influential theorists such as Anthony Giddens, Ulrich Beck and Zygmunt Bauman as part of their descriptions of a major shift from 'modern' societies, came to dominate the intellectual terrain of sociology. While intended initially as a macro level theory of social life, and not primarily addressed to the domain of personal relationships (Smart and Shipman 2004), it has, nevertheless, become a touchstone for discussions on this subject. In relation to the study of personal life, the individualisation thesis made families less important. In brief, an emphasis on agency meant an increased focus on the role of the individual social actor navigating his or her way through the lifecourse. This meant that prescribed roles, such as daughter or husband, were assumed to have less social purchase because they could be defined more creatively than in the past. Of course many sociologists contested the individualisation thesis (Ribbens et al. 2002; Smart 2007) and a number of authors presented trenchant criticisms of the applicability of this concept to the arena of personal relationships by drawing on empirical studies to show that responsibility, obligations, inequality and power relations had not simply disappeared. However, in the wake of this major shift in how to think about contemporary society a continuing focus on family perhaps just seemed rather old fashioned.

There has certainly been a need to reassert that choices do remain structurally constrained; ascribed social relations have not been replaced by 'liquid' relationships which can be remade at will. Yet researchers have also recognised that claims to individualisation had their origins in social changes which have to be taken seriously. Changes which do suggest a degree of transformation – certainly in expectation if less in actuality – around personal and family life. Engaging with the idea of individualisation has therefore led to some interesting developments in the theorising of family life without the wholesale adoption of its argument. This is perhaps easier in theory than in practice. We suggest that if the aim is to develop an understanding of family lives within this mode, the concept of displaying families is useful. As Janet Finch states in her original article, the requirement for family members to display their connection with each other is greater among those who are less recognisable as constituting family (2007: 71). This only makes sense if there are indeed wider social structural contexts (Irwin 2005) which retain importance and influence on how we 'see' family relationships. At the same time, the statement by Finch that display is fundamentally a claim by social agents that '"These are my family relationships, and they work"' (2007: 73) emphasises that this is not a deterministic model where individuals only respond, but instead that they contribute, often intentionally, to how their personal circumstances are read by others. As such the idea of 'displaying family' is a tool which operationalises a fruitful middle way, a socially interactive and dynamic understanding of family life which also acknowledges the ongoing significance of structural contexts.

Challenging 'family': diversity

In recent years a second major concern for the sociology of the family has been how to negotiate (in empirical and theoretical terms) increasing diversity in the organisation of family life. The theme of difference in family forms and living arrangements is associated with the idea of individualisation, in that it is the greater autonomy of individuals over decisions about their personal life which is often posited as the cause. However, thinking about how to conduct and theorise research in the face of a high level of differentiation presents a separate conundrum.

As researchers looked at different household arrangements and networks as defined by those being studied as 'their family', defining what constituted family became increasingly difficult. The recognition that there is no archetypal family which dominates in practice, and perhaps even in ideology, led to 'the family' being replaced by 'families', in similar fashion to the way in which other commonly used sociological categories such as masculinities, femininities and ethnicities were also pluralised. It was explicitly to register that generic definitions about what counted as a family were increasingly meaningless and that a more useful focus was on the practices of family life, that David Morgan (1996) suggested researchers concentrate on the 'doing' rather than the 'being' of family. As Janet Finch says, the concept of 'displaying families' is a direct development of Morgan's family practices, though with a particular focus on the way in which 'the meaning of one's actions has to be both conveyed to and understood by relevant others' (2007: 66). Therefore the idea of 'displaying families' is clearly part of a new tradition, one which offers a way around a previously problematic definitional stalemate.

The concept of 'displaying families' also usefully directs us, as researchers, to what should be studied. The freedom to focus on differences instead of unifying definitions led to an upsurge in detailed studies of the personal lives of groups who had previously been largely ignored. This was justified partly by the 'gap in the literature' argument – that the situation of particular groups who had previously been 'under the radar' of sociologists (at least partially because of a focus on more culturally dominant groups) should now get academic attention. A second justification was that some of these groups deserved attention especially as they had grown in absolute terms and were witnessing greater public attention (for example, stay-at-home fathers). Alongside the 'traditional' social divisions of class, gender and ethnicity, increasing attention was paid to the way in which age and lifecourse stages, sexuality, disability, religious identification, as well as cross-national differences, play a part in influencing our experience of family life. To complicate matters further these dimensions were found to interact and intersect with each other for any individual and within families. Explorations of the way in which these divisions and identities play out have provided interesting data and an insight into the complexity of contemporary family life. However, while disparate studies can provide engaging descriptions there is a risk of conducting studies on particular groups simply because we can, leading to a glut of specific studies whose sociological purpose is unclear. Of course the problem is defining at the outset what is worthy of study and avoiding the reification of existing differences and lines of demarcation: As Gabb (2008: 167) has argued 'suppositions about kinds of families, forms of intimacy and which differences shape behaviour should be resisted'. A focus on practices and display is useful in managing the challenge of deepening our understanding of families and personal relationships while navigating through a wide range of settings and circumstances, as practices and display offer the possibility of moving away from thinking about families in terms of categories which are supposedly, a priori, significant. This focus seems to offer the possibility of a sociology of family life that can reflect, as Jennifer Mason's phrases it, 'the multi-dimensional and vivid nature of real life experience' (2008: 43) rather than reproducing static categories.

Extending and debating the concept of 'displaying families'

In reading through the contributions for this edited collection we were struck by two emergent themes. First, many authors were concerned with the issue of audience. Indeed this was not wholly surprising given that interaction was initially pitched as the unique selling point of 'displaying families' and because Finch gave relatively less attention to the 'to whom' aspect of the question she initially formulated than the 'why'. What emerged from the submissions was that the issue of audience raises issues of reception, negotiation and contestation; that is, who constitutes the audience for display and who controls whether, and the degree to which, an activity is recognised as a display of family. The second theme, which emerged from engagement with how family is displayed and which is explored here through a number of empirical studies as well as more theoretical reflections on the concept, is its expansiveness. While dismissing a structured conception of family in favour of one that is based around practices and therefore the everyday lived reality of family members, the concept does employ the term 'families'. The contributors raised questions as to the extent to which the concept could be – or indeed should be (see Finch's afterword) – extended to include a wider range of personal relationships.

Exploring 'displaying families': the role of audience

Finch's concept is explicitly concerned with interaction because family practices are not 'done' in a social vacuum: it is insufficient for practices associated with family life to be merely carried out; they must also be recognised *as* family practices by others; display is 'the conveying of meanings through social interaction and the acknowledgment of this by relevant others' (Finch 2007: 77). The issues taken up by many of the authors are who counts as 'relevant others' and what counts as 'acknowledgement'; it is perhaps in relation to these issues that there is most disagreement between Janet Finch and those taking up her invitation to explore the concept of 'displaying families' in this volume.

In her original article Finch uses an example from earlier work by Smart and Neale (1999) to illustrate how the 'successful establishment of the family-like nature of relationships is accomplished primarily through direct social interaction with the individuals with whom one is establishing family relationships, who then respond by themselves acting within the framework of those relationships. However, this is reinforced by other participants or observers, who also acknowledge the family-like nature of what they see, hear or learn about' (2007: 74). This has three distinct elements to it. First, display is primarily a direct encounter between those who constitute family. Second, in order to succeed as a display of family it must involve reciprocity. Finally, external others may play a part in confirming the display. It is the latter two aspects which contain some potential ambiguity and which, because of this quality, have been explored in more depth in this volume.

A number of the authors note that Finch's form of words strongly suggests that 'displaying families' only occurs when the practice of display is recognised and received in the way in which it was intended; that is, that this is what marks it out as an effective family practice (Finch 2007: 67). Our interpretation is that Finch, in her original article, is focusing on delineating what are displays of *family* versus practices that could be considered displays of something else. Some authors in this collection have noted, however, that a display of family relations still exists even if it is not reciprocated. Further, they argue that it may be especially worthwhile to explore *when* displays are misrecognised or simply not accepted by others because these, as well as 'successful' displays, provide an important lens for understanding the boundaries of what constitutes family relations. Using Smart and Neale (1999) Finch cites the example of a divorced father who reinvents his parenting practice in order to engage with his children in a new set of circumstances and who is praised for this adaptation by his ex-mother-in-law; she says that he is a good father. However, it is equally possible to envisage an alternative scenario, whereby this shift in parenting style is not interpreted as a positive display of fatherhood that reinforces his family relationships, but is instead categorised as a display of something else, such as a display of power over his ex-wife. In this alternative example of post-divorce parenting a father has had *no* recognition of his efforts to be an involved parent, despite his attempts; in other words, his display of family has been unsuccessful. However, as sociologists, surely we would wish to argue that unsuccessful display still provides us with something of value for understanding family relations.

Finch emphasises in her afterword that display 'is not only about conveying meaning to external agencies, or seeking reactions in a public context' but that it is as much about 'conveying social meaning *to each other*' (Chapter 11, original emphasis): this aspect of display does indeed merit underlining. However, it is the complexity of the range of participants and possible mismatch of responses which provoked the most interest from contributors. This is perhaps most marked in relation to the role of 'external others'. Many of the authors here (including Haynes and Dermott, Seymour, and McIntosh and colleagues) reflect on the existence of multiple potential audiences.

Finch suggests that some of these reflections on the role of those out-side the immediate network of family relationships conflates observing display with experiencing display – 'where there are criticisms of the concept of display authors tend to be writing about the process of *observing* display' (Chapter 11, original emphasis). It is certainly true that in some instances external actors may be simply observers and as such their view on a particular practice may not be relevant to its status as a display of family relations for the direct participants. Recognising this is important in order to avoid spreading the net too widely in defining *relevant others*. Yet, it also seems to us that external individuals and groups of people may constitute the direct audience for display; they are, in other words, participants in the creation of 'displaying families'. For example, a couple wishing to adopt have to 'display' their credentials as a possible family unit to an adoption agency. In this instance the need for reciprocity from an organisation that is external to family members themselves defines a powerful external individual or group as a participant in the construction of display, not merely as an observer.

Beyond displaying families': 'displaying personal relationships'?

It has already been noted that the term 'family' has, for some considerable time, been rejected as inadequate for conveying the multiplicities inherent in family life. Even when pluralised to 'families' the term is still insufficient to cover the range of relationships which those traditionally branded sociologists of family life wish to examine. To include the wider relationships and negotiations that take place with friends, partners, acquaintances and colleagues along with those we call 'family' (whether that is defined as close biological kin or a looser definition), it has become commonplace to refer to 'personal lives', 'personal relationships' or the study of 'intimacy' as terms which encompass, but are not restricted to, the narrower 'family'. While we might be tempted to dismiss these variations as mere semantics, debates over terminology, as Carol Smart suggests in her book titled *Personal Life* (2007), are significant because they reflect conceptual shifts and empirical changes. The current discussions in this area therefore indicate how the field is 'going through a very interesting phrase as the sociological imagination stretches and reconfigures in order better to grasp and reflect the complexities of contemporary personal life' (Smart 2007: 27). This interest in reflecting on what choices of terminology mean in relation to what we study and how we conceptualise our field of research is evident directly and indirectly in the contributions included in this collection.

Responding to Brian Heaphy's (Chapter 2) query about the decision to restrict the concept to 'displaying *families*' and his concomitant suggestion that its applicability to other social relationships deserves attention, Janet Finch – in her afterword – reasserts that her starting point was the idea of *family* practices, understanding the term as 'sets of activities involving specific individuals, which take on social meaning associated with "family"' (Chapter 11). Therefore, in developing 'doing family' and making a case for the concept of 'displaying families' she intentionally focussed solely on families. Intriguingly though, she nevertheless does not rule out the possibility of an extension of display to other kinds of relationships. She does state, however, that any translation into the broader arena of personal relationships would not necessarily be straightforward because, although commonalities would exist, this development would require not only further, but different, thinking. We think that it is worthwhile to ponder this possibility a little more.

Although 'family' was criticised as too restrictive because it implies a normative family type that can be relatively easily delineated and therefore positions many people's experiences of family as outside of this, at the same time it is a word which continues to be understood in everyday language and that alone gives it some value. It is perhaps because of this commonsense appeal that, although challenged and explored as problematic, the word has not been entirely dismissed from the lexicon; more often than not it is added to, hence 'families and relationships' or 'intimacy and family life'. Family as negotiated, complicated and even contested makes sense to us as individuals.

Would it be possible to replace 'displaying families' with 'displaying intimacy'? We are not convinced that this would be a good route. Intimacy has had a strong association with individualisation (after Giddens 1992) and in everyday usage has connotations of sexual relations. Sociology generally adopts something akin to Lynn Jamieson's useful description of intimacy as 'representing a very particular kind of "closeness" and being "special" to another person founded on self-disclosure ... characterised by knowledge and understanding' (Jamieson 2005: 2411) which plays down any sexual element. However, this is not the case with other disciplines that are also concerned with the subject area; for example, in one recent textbook on intimate relationships (Bradbury and Karney 2010), the authors define their scope at the outset; an intimate relationship is certainly more than just sex requiring 'strong, sustained mutual influence' (Bradbury and Karney 2010: 11) but, in their definition, it does also feature 'at least the *potential* for sexual interaction' (Bradbury and Karney 2010: 11, our emphasis). However, the more significant reason for not using the term 'displaying intimacy' is that the idea of display is fundamentally about the acknowledgement of social relations and the 'display' is about the existence of a relationship, rather than the *quality* which is at the heart of the term intimacy. What we feel is of particular importance to Finch is that 'displaying family' should emphasise a focus on defining the contours of 'my family' to others. As various authors in this collection have mentioned, the requirement to display family may involve a wide range of potential audiences that are not restricted to family members including, for example, researchers (Kehily and Thomson, Chapter 4) and abstract participants such as the state (Haynes and Dermott, Chapter 8). Some settings may require a simultaneous display for 'family' and 'non-family' members (Seymour, Chapter 9 and McIntosh and colleagues, Chapter 10). Yet, for the most part practices of display are centred on those in close social proximity and/or direct contact, such as the negotiations with their own parents in Almack's account of lesbian mothers (Chapter 6). The term 'family' is important to individuals and, especially when 'the contours of "my family" are not necessarily obvious or easy to identify' (Finch 2007: 70), there is a need to display it. Individuals are saying specifically that 'this is my family and it works' and not that these are 'just' important social relationships to me.

The label 'displaying family/ies' does seem to be the most appropriate term to apply to Finch's specific definition. However, the question whether there is any usefulness in extending the term to other kinds of relationships still stands. A useful corollary for exploring this is the idea of 'displaying friends'. An initial attempt at thinking through this comparison between 'displaying families' and 'displaying friends' suggests strong similarities between them based on the ways in which 'displaying families' has been discussed by the authors in this collection and by Finch herself. 'Displaying friends' could also be thought of as becoming more pertinent at particular moments in time, having various audiences, and being more acute for particular groups who may not so easily 'look' from the outside as friends. We might think about moments in time when friendship needs to be displayed or is expected to be displayed, such as at times of emotional or material trauma like a bereavement, or when happy life events occur like the birth of a child. We could also note that boundaries between friend and non-friend are often blurred and that practices may need to be more overt in order to assert to an audience that 'this is my friend', as a specific display perhaps among groups of children within a school. Similarly there may be a need to negatively display, that there is 'only' a friendship rather than a sexual relationship between a single heterosexual man and single heterosexual woman. There are more options that could also be explored, such as how there could be a mismatch between the intention of a display of friendship and how it is received. To suggest that this extension is viable and potentially useful does not mean that it can necessarily be stretched further to include all social relationships; the acquaintanceships, for example, that are the subject of a recent book by Morgan (2009) would seem to fit less well under the rubric of 'display'. There is also perhaps the need to explore further the extent to which 'display' can be extended to include other, not explicitly family, 'practices' (an issue which Seymour raises in her chapter in this volume). However, it is our belief that part of the appeal and value of the idea of 'displaying families' is precisely because it does have a broader applicability. Speculating about how extending the concept outwards would be of value involves considering whether 'displaying personal relationships' has any use or sociological resonance, a question we leave the readers of this volume to reflect upon. In conclusion we turn to another writer on family relationships. Janet Carsten has written that kinship is 'an area of life in which people invest their emotions, their creative energy, and their new imaginings' (2004: 9); our hope is that this volume marks the beginning of a new discussion about how best to research and understand the important and complex world of contemporary family life.

2
Critical Relational Displays

Brian Heaphy

Introduction

In her original article on the topic Janet Finch (2007) proposes that 'display' can extend our understandings of contemporary family practices. Display, she argues, is a characteristic activity of contemporary families, and it is an idea that can usefully be added to the conceptual toolbox for analysing these. Finch invites researchers to debate and refine the concept of family display, and I take up this invitation to evaluate its potential contribution to a critical and reflexive sociology of contemporary relational life. In doing so, I concentrate on the ways in which the concept could be refined to address the situated significance of display as an activity for different kinds of families and relationships; the links between display and the power and politics of contemporary relational life; and how display is bound up with the performativity and scripting of family and 'other' relationships.

Finch's emphasis is on the distinctive significance of display for contemporary families. While displays should be historically located, we should also consider the other ways in which they are situated. One way of doing this is to reflect on the different significance of display to diverse *families*. Finch argues that families increasingly *need* displaying. However, this need is not merely the result of family change, diversity and fluidity. Critically, we should interrogate if the need to display family applies more to some social constituencies in specific contexts than others. We should also ask what the requirement to display reveals about the flow of power with respect to relational life. Reflexively, we should ask how the sociology of display might be located with respect to the politics of relational life. Finch suggests that reflexive agency and social interactions are crucial to family display. I agree, but this is only part of the story. As sociologists, we should also critically and reflexively consider how display is linked to the performativity of family and 'other' relational forms. This can enable an understanding of how the reflexive scripting of display is constrained, and how the relational practices and interactions involved in displaying are linked to family structures and institutions. It also points to the potential dangers of sociological discourse about family display that confirms family privilege and sidelines 'other' relational displays. The critical-reflexive incorporation of display into our analyses of contemporary relationships can enhance our situated sociological understandings of both family and display.

Structure and argument

This chapter begins by situating Finch's understanding of family display with respect to its sociological influences. Display is linked to ideas about doing family, family practices and reflexive relating that have shaped British family studies in the last decade or so. It combines themes in Finch's previous work with Morgan's arguments about family practices, theoretical arguments about the reflexivity of contemporary relational life and the findings of British empirical studies about family diversity and fluidity. Thus, display develops a new dimension of the *sociology of contemporary reflexive family practices*, and offers a new tool for investigating their multi-dimensionality. Distinguishing between this sociology and the *reflexive sociology of family and relating*, I suggest that the value of display to the latter is also worth considering.

Following this I consider the significance of family diversity and difference to this second area of focus; that is, the reflexive sociology of family display. This shifts the emphasis away from display as increasingly necessary in historical terms to the different ways it is important across and within diverse families. Demands to display, and investments in it, are likely to vary for different kinds of families: couple and lone parent, middle and working class, white and ethnic minority, heterosexual and lesbian and gay and so on. Demands and investments are also likely to vary within families, especially for women and men. In these ways and others, display is linked to the power and politics of relational life, and the next section of this chapter makes these links explicit. Family displaying is linked to power in that it involves making family claims that are more or less readily recognised and validated according to how relationships approximate the interlinked cultural ideals of 'normal', 'proper' and 'good' families. Family displays are political because they are linked to inclusions and exclusions from relational citizenship.

The following section discusses in more detail such power and politics by considering the 'necessities' of family display and linking them to the performativities of family and 'other' relationships. Viewed performatively, displaying is intimately linked to reproducing family as an institution, and to power*ful* discursive frames and meaning systems through which relationships are constructed, given meaning, legitimated and 'othered'. While a performative view of display highlights family and relational constraints, display also involves critical, resistive and creative operations of power. The multi-dimensionality of power with respect to relational displays can be illuminated through consideration of how they are scripted. In conclusion I argue that a critical and reflexive sociology of family would interrogate its own assumptions about and orientation towards *family* scripting.

Situating family display as a sociological concept

Finch's ideas about family display are rooted first and foremost in interconnected sociological ideas about 'doing family' and 'family practices'. These emphasise the social and relational practices through which families are (re)produced: family is defined less by 'blood' or legal ties and more by activities culturally deemed family. 'Doing family' perspectives explore families as *social* projects or achievements. They are concerned with how families are actually lived, and the active part their participants play in shaping them. They often attempt to put aside normative questions about how families *should* be organised.

Finch's own work on family responsibilities illuminates the sociological insights of the doing family approach. Through studying how family responsibilities are done, Finch and Mason's (1993) research troubled the normative idea that family membership implies binding relational obligations. They found that, in practice, adult family responsibilities were based on negotiated commitments that were actively worked out over time. Their study suggested that: '[t]hrough negotiation people create sets of material and moral baggage which gets carried forward, and which help create the framework for future negotiations' (Finch and Mason 1993: 92–3). Through doing family (or not), adult relatives negotiate their commitments to each other. For example, if siblings discontinue doing family with each other they can effectively cease to be family in practice, and are likely to feel less responsible for each other over time. Thus, the doing family approach also recognises family contingency. Finch draws on Morgan's (1996) ideas about family practice to link the doing of family to family display:

> The starting point for this analysis [of family display] is the recognition that contemporary families are defined more by 'doing' family things than by 'being' a family. The most influential discussion of this is Morgan's (1996) work on family practices, which radically shifts sociological analysis away from 'family' as a structure … towards understanding families as sets of activities which take on a particular meaning, associated with family, at a given point in time. 'Family' is a facet of social life, not a social institution, it 'represents a quality rather than a thing'. (2007: 62)

As Finch notes, the family practice frame considers family to be irreducible to household and biological or legal kin. Rather, Finch states, it focuses on practices that are given meaning *as* family practices by their location in cultural systems of meaning, and 'itself incorporates a number of key concepts which other scholars have used to analyze contemporary families – fluidity, diversity, multi-facetedness' (Finch 2007: 66). Finch draws on these ideas to argue that displaying has become an especially significant aspect of practice because of the increasingly contingent, fluid and diverse nature of family.

In recent years the openness and dynamism of family has been illuminated by a number of empirical studies of how families are 'done' in and through practice. Finch illustrates her argument about the increasing need to display family by referencing studies of family practices post-divorce (Smart and Neale 1999), inheritance practices (Finch and Mason 2000), lesbian and gay family practices (Weeks et al. 2001) and other dimensions of contemporary family life (Ribbens McCarthy et al. 2003; Williams 2004). Contrary to culturally pessimistic and politically conservative arguments about the demise of 'the family', these studies illuminate how family as practice is alive and well amongst what Finch terms conventional and unconventional families. In fact, people nowadays appear to display strong commitments to family whether or not their relationships correspond to conventional family forms.

Viewed through the lens of family practices and display, the differences between families seem less important than their commonalities. While divorced, reconstituted and lesbian and gay families might still be viewed as 'unconventional' family forms, research suggests their participants are engaged in very *ordinary* family activities. Nowadays, Finch suggests, display is a very ordinary requirement of 'all' families as a means of claiming 'this is my family and it works' (2007: 70). Summarizing the empirical evidence for both conventional and unconventional family forms, Finch states:

> Relationships need to be worked at in order to be sustained, and this is apparently done with a sense of real commitment which will necessarily
>
> entail actively demonstrating that a former partner, or the step child of
>
> one's son, or a close friend, is indeed part of that set of relationships which one regards as family relationships, and that family relationships thus configured do really 'work'. (2007: 70)

The increased need for display as the active demonstration of commitment is linked to the historically distinctive nature of contemporary family dynamism and contingency. For Finch, this implies social actors' cognizance of the interlinked need for displaying and claiming family: 'the recognition that relationships are fluid, that they have changed and will change again, underpins the need to demonstrate that "my current family relationships" really work well, however little they resemble those of other people' (2007: 70). Thus framed, Finch's arguments echo late modern theoretical propositions about transforming relational forms and their implications for self-reflexivity. Indeed, she argues:

> The third reason why display is important in contemporary families is the link to personal identity, itself an important feature of much recent research on family life. The influential work of Giddens, Beck, Beck-Gernsheim and others on the construction of identities in late modern societies (Beck, 1992; Beck and Beck Gernsheim, 1995; Giddens, 1991) has highlighted the link both between relationships and social processes, and between interpersonal intimacy and personal identity. The implication is that intimate relationships are subject to change as the individual identities which they support (or no longer support) are also changing. This adds a further level of fluidity to contemporary family relationships and reinforces the need to display those relationships which are meaningful at any given point in time. (2007: 70)

Thus situated, Finch's argument about display develops an overlooked dimension of contemporary *reflexive* family practices. Reflexivity has numerous meanings. In Giddens's sense it implies self-consciousness about self and relational openness that promotes efforts to negotiate commitments and make them explicit. In Beck and Beck-Gernsheim's sense, it implies a reflex response to the risks associated with self and relational openness. This can lead to intimate conflicts as people are subjected to pressures to self-realise that are in tension with commitments to each other. While these reflexivity arguments have influenced recent sociological understandings of contemporary family practices, they have also been subjected to trenchant criticism. Critics argue that they overplay the agency, choices and 'freedoms' that people have with respect to how they can relate, and underplay continuities with respect to how relating practices are institutionalised, structured along axes of differences and linked to the flow of power (for example, Jamieson 1998).

Drawing on these criticisms, I have argued elsewhere a major weakness of theorising about *reflexive relating* is its failure to interrogate its *own* normative and 'political' orientations (Heaphy 2007). Put another way, the sociology of reflexive relating tends towards being an *unreflexive* sociology. On the one hand, it uncritically expounds contestable claims about the 'reflexive making' of contemporary intimate relationships. On the other hand, it fails to incorporate critical sociological work on family life (from Marxian, feminist, structuralist, post-structuralist and psychoanalytic perspectives) that would trouble these claims (see Heaphy 2007). Arguments about relational reflexivity are partial in the sense that they only tell part of the story about contemporary relational life (that people engage in their relationships in a self-conscious and 'knowing' way), and also in that they are not 'neutral' with respect to normative claims (they conflate the idea that people *should* be self-conscious and knowing with the claim that they *are*).

Because of these partial and normative influences, the concept of display risks being uncritically orientated towards the sociology of reflexive family relating. To counter this, it is worthwhile asking if it could also contribute to a different kind of sociology: a *reflexive sociology* of family and relating. Reflexive sociology, like reflexivity, has many meanings and there are competing models for doing reflexive sociology (Lynch 2000). I use the term loosely to describe 'self-critical' approaches to sociological analysis where scholars are collectively willing to: interrogate and trouble their own assumptions, and where the burden is not on the auto-reflexivity of the individual researcher (Adkins 2002; Bourdieu and Wacquant 1992); acknowledge that sociological knowledge is implicated in the flow of power, especially where propositions about social reality are concerned (Steier 1991); and accept that expert claims (including sociological ones) should be explored for their normative orientations, inclusions and exclusions, and the ways in which they support operations of power with respect to difference and inequality (Ramazanoglu and Holland 2002). In the following sections it is my aim to debate and refine the concept of display in a way that shifts the ground of discussion towards this critical and reflexive sociology of family and relating. Thus, by concentrating on issues of difference, power and performativity I am focusing as much on 'displaying *families*' as on '*displaying* families'.

Display, diversity and difference

What are the implications of diversity and difference for the critical-reflexive sociology of family display, and how is display significant in different ways across and within families? Finch argues that family diversity influences the need to display family, but only briefly mentions variations in how families are required to display. Different requirements and investments with respect to displaying *within* families are not remarked upon. A fuller incorporation of diversity and difference into our thinking would better equip us to conceptualise displays as socio-culturally situated.

Different 'demands' to display across families can be illuminated by consideration of the axes along which family diversity is most often discussed in contemporary sociology: social class, ethnicity, lone parenting and sexuality. Working-class and middle-class families are likely to be invested in display. However, they are likely to be subjected to different demands and investments with respect to it. Respectable family display has been linked to moral and economic rectitude since the nineteenth century through its association with bourgeois norms and values and middle-class constructions of family. Modern family ideals as construed in expert, policy and political discourse were modelled on such constructions and were central to modern relational governance. Class theorists viewed this construction of family as supporting the needs of modern capitalism, feminists argued that it supported the modern patriarchal order, and Foucauldians linked it to Panoptical surveillance and governance. Theoretically, late modernity is associated with post-Panoptical freedom. However, as Bauman (2000) argues, those at the bottom of social hierarchies continue to be subjected to intense surveillance.

It is worth asking if families at the lower end of class hierarchies are still the most likely to be closely monitored by state agencies. If so, they are more likely than middle-class families to be subjected to intense demands to monitor their relational displays in line with social requirements. Given that 'proper', 'good' and 'successful' families are still measured in accordance with the norms, practices and 'relational habitus' (cf. Bourdieu 1977; Bourdieu and Wacquant 1992) of well-resourced, middle-class families, middle-class constituencies are predisposed to 'successful' display and working-class families to being judged as 'failing'. While late modernity opens up some opportunities to experiment with relating, we should remember Bauman's additional point that the consequences of failed experiments are likely to be greater for those at the bottom of class hierarchies. Limited resources constrain access to second chances. In this respect, working-class failures to display families 'properly' (and conventionally) can have high costs and irredeemable consequences (for example, when parents are deemed to be failing and children are taken into care).

The need for display is also likely to cut across ethnically diverse families. However, the resources, norms, practices and relational habitus of *white* middle-class families have historically been the benchmark against which successful families and displays of these are measured. Black families continue to be constructed as problematic and culturally 'strange'. For example, discourse about the lack of male role models in African-Caribbean families construct black families as failing, as does discourse about the failure of Asian families to integrate. Simultaneously, poor white families are constructed as 'other' to cosmopolitanism, as are 'radicalising' Muslim families. On the one hand, there is some cultural acceptance of the *fact* of family diversity. On the other hand, the practices of black, Muslim and poor white families are construed as 'other' to the extent that they deviate from white middle-class norms. The white middle-class family is the standard of 'proper' and 'good' display. Those who are neither white nor middle class are predisposed to being judged as failing to display appropriately.

The risks of being judged as failing to display family appropriately are especially high for lone-parent families. In this case class, gender, ethnicity and age are combined with family form in constructions of feckless mothers, absent fathers and irresponsible single-parent families who 'sponge' on the state. Moral panics about single-parent families have gendered, classed and 'raced' dimensions. They are underpinned by concerns about unpartnered, young working-class women who fail to display their subscription to white middle-class norms of 'responsible' relating. The demands and incentives to display 'respectable' lone-parent families are high, but the strength of popular and political discourse about the failures of black or white working-class mothers predisposes such displays to being judged as inadequate. While it *is* possible nowadays to display forms of respectable lone-parent families – for example, post-divorce – this is largely dependent on embodying privileged relational habitus.

The relational displays of working-class, black and lone-parent families are likely to be constructed as evidence of deviant families to the extent that they do not conform to white middle-class family practice *and* form. Where does this leave lesbian, gay or queer families? Research supports late modern theoretical arguments that these are highly reflexive. Lesbian, gay and queer families tend to be highly conscious of how they do and display family, especially where children are involved. This is partly because their relationships are often constructed as especially risky (see Weeks et al. 2001). While lesbian and gay families have become more 'acceptable' and 'respectable' in recent decades, some theory and research suggest that this has been conditional on adopting and displaying white middle-class heterosexual norms (Taylor 2009). On the one hand, research indicates that lesbian and gay displays of family are bound up with claims to relational citizenship. On the other hand, it suggests that in day-to-day contexts lesbian and gay families are still often denied recognition by virtue of displaying the 'wrong' family form (Heaphy and Yip 2006). There remain social and legal penalties for not displaying families properly (see Klesse 2007; Smith 1997). Indeed, several theorists argue that this explains why same-sex marriage and civil unions have been embraced by many lesbians and gay men. Arrangements like Civil Partnership impose a model of respectability on same-sex relationships that is dependent upon displaying conformity to the highest 'standard' of the white middle-class family: marriage. Simultaneously, Civil Partnership retains 'real' marriage as a privilege for heterosexual families.

The links between frames for displaying family and social governance are also evident in different demands and investments in display *within* families. One detailed example will suffice to illustrate this: gender. There is a wealth of feminist work on how doing family is linked to doing gender (see Cranny-Francis et al. 2003). Put another way, men and women are socially orientated towards different displaying practices, and family display is thus bound up with the (re)production of gender inequalities. Studies of the unequal division of labour within heterosexual families suggest that women are socially orientated towards doing the bulk of socially and economically undervalued domestic tasks like feeding, cleaning, shopping and caring, because these are tied to conceptions about the proper doing and displaying of femininity (Delphy and Leonard 1992). In this respect, the display of family and of femininity is intertwined. While heterosexual men invest in family display, some research suggests that they are more likely to be socially orientated towards displaying 'the picture' but less to doing the low valued tasks and emotion work that making the picture involves (Duncombe and Marsden 1999).

Family display and emotion work are likely to be interconnected, and a number of studies suggest that women more than men are socially orientated towards doing emotion work within heterosexual relationships (Duncombe and Marsden 1999). Emotion work is linked to display in two obvious ways. First, there is the work involved in managing one's own emotions and in displaying the right kind of family and gendered family 'role' (wife/husband). Second, there is the work involved in displaying love and commitment by caring for others. The evidence is that women are more likely to do the bulk of such emotion and displaying work. Many aspects of displaying family, from remembering and marking special occasions to performing domestic and caring tasks, are culturally deemed to be women's work. A critically reflexive sociology of family display would therefore consider how displaying work is gendered and linked to gendered inequalities.

Diverse displays, power and politics

How differences matter in structuring requirements to display is linked to how diverse family and relational forms are situated in terms of the power and the politics of display. It was noted earlier that Finch links display to how families are historically situated and to contemporary claims that 'this is my family and it works'. But as we have seen, families are also situated in other ways and family diversity is especially important in this respect. Finch acknowledges family differences in some ways, but does not fully draw out their implications for display or its links to power and politics. Acknowledging diversity she notes that '[a]ll recent influential empirical work on contemporary families emphasises the essential diversity of family composition' (2007: 67), and that family form can influence the need to display:

> [The] diversity and fluidity of contemporary family relationships are core reasons why displaying families is necessary. Does this mean that displaying families is important only in those situations where relationships take a non-conventional form? ...it seems very likely that the need for display is greater as relationships move

further away from those which are readily recognizable as constituting family relationships. (2007: 71)

Diversity, for Finch, is a matter of the range of 'conventional' and 'non-conventional' relational forms that are nowadays claimed as family. While she acknowledges that display may be a greater requirement for families that do not match conventional forms, she emphasises that to focus only on this would be to 'miss a central point of display':

> In a world where families are defined by the qualitative character of the relationships rather than by membership, and where individual identities are deeply bound up with those relationships, *all* relationships require an element of display to sustain them as family relationships. (2007: 71)

The argument that display cuts across diversity is convincing when viewed through the lenses of arguments about contemporary relational reflexivity as discussed earlier. Relational reflexivity arguments imply that 'all' contemporary families are unconventional when compared to 'traditional' families, and this logic supports the view that 'all' families require displaying. However, it is important not to underplay the qualitative point that different displaying 'requirements' are linked to the power and politics of family life. The different extents to which display is required are linked to the ways in which diverse relational forms are culturally construed as non-normative and how specific displaying requirements are politically and socio-culturally located.

Family displaying is intimately bound up with *claiming* family, but some claims are more immediately validated than others. Some actors are more readily recognised and legitimated as family actors than others. Similarly, some relationships are more likely to be recognised as families than others, and validated as thus. Also, some relational displays are more easily accepted as family displays in the mainstream culture. Invariably it is those actors and relationships that most closely approximate the cultural ideals of 'normal' families, as described in the previous section, whose displays are most likely to be recognised, validated and legitimated. Thus, display as a claim to recognition is not wholly separable from conceptions of 'proper' families which, in turn, are closely connected to conceptions of morally and socially 'good' families.

Family displays are political because they are linked to inclusions and exclusions from relational 'citizenship' (cf. Berlant 1997; Plummer 2003; Weeks et al. 2001). The relational citizenship is not only a matter of being legally recognised *as* family, important as it is, but about the legal, social and cultural recognition afforded relational forms on their own terms, including those that are not family. It is worth asking if *family* is something that *must* be displayed to be fully recognised as relational citizens, and to avoid relationships being defined (and dismissed) as less valid or important. While some 'unconventional' families and relationships may nowadays be recognised as legitimate, we should acknowledge how the acceptable limits of unconventionality are legally, socially and culturally drawn and, as well, the axes of difference and (dis)advantage along which they are drawn. We should recognise that, as illuminated in the previous section, these limits shape the *kinds* of displays that are demanded for relationships to be recognised as 'proper', 'good' and 'valued'.

A critical and reflexive sociology of display would consider all family displays and practices as 'anthropologically strange' and question how people are encouraged or incited to practice and display families and relationships in specific ways. In doing this, it could be seen that, while there may be greater acceptance of family diversity and 'unconventionality' nowadays, the boundaries and frames – or shared meaning systems – that shape family practices and displays have not shifted so much that they have become radically open. These boundaries and frames are also bound up with the regulation of family and relational life and this, as well as the connections between the sociological narration of display and power and politics, can be illuminated via discussion of the performativities and scripting of display.

The performativities and scripting of display

Finch (2007: 73) proposes that in analysing displays we should concern ourselves with social interaction. Analysing displays as situated interactions raises the following kinds of questions: *Who* is claiming recognition for the family-like quality of their relationships and whose recognition is sought?; *How* are claims for recognition conveyed, received and responded to?; and *Where* and *when* are specific kinds of claims conveyed, received and responded to? These questions highlight display as temporally and spatially located interaction. As discussed in the previous sections, display also involves socio-culturally and politically situated interaction. A critical sociology would interrogate the links between complexly situated displaying interactions and flows of power. A reflexive sociology would, in addition, interrogate how its own claims about displaying interaction are linked to this flow. The following discussion considers how arguments about performativity and scripting can help to frame critical-reflexive analyses of displaying interactions.

Display and performativity

In line with its social interactionist rooting, display is constitutive of family and relational experience and not merely reflective of it. The logic of Finch's argument proposes that display constitutes family in line with existing frameworks of meaning. In other words, display is necessarily influenced by dominant frameworks through which families and exclusions from it are defined. Direct connections can be made between the concepts of display and performativity. A performative view of family display would interrogate how it is interconnected with relational governance, the reproduction of family as a privileged relational form, and how inclusions and exclusions from family are linked to reproducing relational inequalities.

To view relational display performatively is to acknowledge its links to power, as family is a hegemonic discursive configuration through which relationships are legitimated, regulated and 'othered'. In Britain and elsewhere, family is institutionally supported and culturally inscribed as *the* legitimate relational form within hierarchies of relationships. It is powerful because it is the frame through which relationships tend to be viewed, and the standard against which their value is often judged. Recognition as family, and successful claims to it, allow access to legal, socio-cultural and economic benefits that come with full relational citizenship such as state sponsored financial and social supports; immigration, adoption and parenting rights; community and expert supports; representational rights and so on.

Family recognition is a *privilege*, and to be constructed as 'other' to family implies compromised relational citizenship. This is especially evident in how, in Britain in the 1980s, constructions of 'pretend family relationships' were central to the denial of full relational citizenship for lesbian and gay men (Weeks et al. 2001). Not every relationship is allowed recognition as family, or is validated as equal to family. However, there are powerful incentives to claim recognition as family because of the access it affords to full relational citizenship. For those relationships that display the 'natural' traits of families, full relational recognition and citizenship can seem like a freely given right. Those relationships that fail to display 'normal' family characteristics are likely to be constructed as second class families or as 'other' to family. As discussed earlier, notions of natural and normal families have historically tended to be equated with white, middle-class, heterosexual relational forms.

Finch dismisses the relevance of performativity to analysing display on the basis that 'in the influential work of Judith Butler ... performativity has more to do with individual identity than with the nature of social interactions' (2007: 76). However, this underplays how performativity is essentially a relational concept and, like social interactionism, is concerned with practice and meaning frames as mutually implicated. Both approaches are concerned with the influence of embodied practice on meaning, and the influence of meaning frames on embodied practice. Also, the concept of performativity can be applied to relationships as much as it can to identity. Indeed, Austin's (1962) original discussion of the concept illuminated it via the example of marriage. There are, however, two interlinked ways in which performativity is orientated towards a different kind of analysis than social interactionism as Finch discusses it. The concept of performativity is more *explicitly* concerned with operations of power as they concern the normative dimensions of discourse and interaction. The concept speaks more directly to the need to interrogate how dominant frames of meaning shape *and* sanction social actions and practices as legitimate. Second, performativity is not only concerned with how relational practices are shaped by the dominating culture, but suggests that our most intimate and relational desires are produced through it. The latter insight is one of performativity's strengths as a concept. It is also, however, one of its weaknesses: it is often deemed to inadequately address creative agency.

In contrast to performativity, display seems more conducive to incorporating living, creative and *knowing* people as is clear where, as Finch argues, display is linked to the claim 'this is my family and it works'. On closer inspection, however, this claim is itself *normatively* framed as it prioritises a claim to family over other relationships (for example, friendship, community, partnerships and so on). It is not simply a claim about the quality of a relationship (for example, that it involves love, commitment, care and so on) but a claim to the privileged relationship 'family'. Indeed, the emphasis that Finch places on this statement in explaining the 'need' for display itself points to how dominating the cultural formation 'family' is as a normative frame. This prompts an obvious question: why is there such an embedded and enduring need to claim recognition and legitimation *as family?*

In contrast to Finch's proposition outlined earlier that such 'need' stems from reflexive recognition of the increasingly 'open' nature of family life, the performative view would link it to family's status as a culturally privileged fiction: family is a powerful story that cultures tell about relationalities that matter most. Family is so 'naturalised' and taken for granted that its discursive and fictive nature very easily slips away from view. Its effectiveness as a form of relational governance is evidenced in how difficult it is for relational practices and displays to escape being viewed through the family frame: *as* family or not. A critical-reflexive sociology of family could incorporate the performative by asking the following question: Is family *so* dominating as a cultural frame that sociologists themselves are orientated towards imposing the categories of 'family' or 'not family' on the range of relational practices and displays they observe and encounter? This raises the issue of how relationships and displays are scripted *as* family ones in day-to-day life and sociologically.

Scripting display

In highlighting the links between display and performativity I am not proposing that we should reject display in favour of a performative view of relationships. One of the strengths of display as a concept is that it acknowledges change and agency with respect to family life in a way that performativity does not. One of the weaknesses of performativity as a concept is that it risks over-emphasising the circularity of power or its disciplinary dimensions and undermining critical, resistive and creative displays and operations of power. The challenge, as I see it, is to think about the ways in which display could be better informed by the critical concerns at the heart of concept of performativity, whilst acknowledging the latter's limitations.

One way of bridging social interactionist and performative frames in analysing the multi-dimensionality of power with respect to relational display, is to focus on how the latter is *scripted*. In the past, scripting has been associated with a kind of symbolic interactionism that was concerned with how social actions and interaction follow scripts. This is an impoverished view of scripting theory, and as Plummer argues about sexual scripting theory:

> In the hands of some researchers, it [scripting theory] has become a wooden mechanical tool for identifying uniformities in [] conduct: the script determines activity, rather than emerging though activity. What is actually required is to show the nature of [] scripts as they *emerge* in encounters. (Plummer, quoted in Knapp Whittier and Melendez 2004: 132)

Drawing from interactionist principles (see Gagnon 1990; Knapp Whittier and Melendez 2004; Longmore 1998; Simon and Gagnon 1986, 2003 for discussions of these with respect to sexual relations), scripting can be deployed as an analytical tool for thinking about how displays are linked to family discourse at a cultural level, the 'naturalised' meanings and practices that people bring to their relationships, and how through *interaction* in relationships 'new' relationship stories emerge. These discourses, naturalised meanings and practices and stories can be conceptualised as interlinked orders of relational scripting that influence and are influenced by display. Analysing these at an experiential level entails exploring how *habituated personal scripts* for relational displaying are influenced by *cultural scripts* about family, but also how interlinked habituated and cultural scripts are resisted, altered, troubled and transformed *through* interactions. On the one hand, it would be naive to ignore the significance and power of relational scripting at the level of culture and habituated practice. Family displays always reference such scripting. On the other hand, it would be equally naive to ignore how new relational scripts at the level of culture and personal practice could emerge through interaction. To explore relational displays as scripted is to acknowledge that they are neither wholly given nor wholly creative. Rather, it is to acknowledge that they are both 'given' *and* dynamic. It is also a way of acknowledging continuities and changes in how families are displayed, and that the flow of power with respect to display is not uni-directional: family displaying is not only creative or constraining; it is both.

Analytically, attention to the reflexive scripting of display needs to be combined with attention to the less reflexive and more habituated ways in which displays are scripted. Even the most reflexive and self-conscious family displays will be influenced by 'naturalised' habits and desires. Not to recognise this is to steer too close to a kind of sociology of reflexive family and relating that overemphasises change, agency and creativity. Interpretation is the key issue here. We should focus on how relational displays are interpreted and given meaning in day-to-day living, and collectively also take a reflexive step back to ask how hegemonic cultural scripts shape our sociological interpretations of these displays and their significance. Studying relational displays as scripted thus entails critically addressing our own normative assumptions about the stories that relational displays tell, and our orientations towards sociologically scripting these. In an era of radically diverse relational practices (such as those detailed in the empirical work discussed earlier), the fact that family remains the dominating frame for sociologically interpreting and scripting relationships speaks volumes about the power of the family imaginary and the need for a more critical orientation to it.

Conclusion: scripting critical relational displays

In discussing display, Finch implies that family displaying has become a critically important activity because nowadays family is no longer simply given. Increasingly it is something we 'all' have to claim. In debating the concept in the way that I have, my aim has been to argue the case for the situated and critical study of relational display. This would acknowledge the different ways in which family display is critical for diverse families, and that *family* display is critical because of the privileged position of family with respect to relational citizenship. Thus, family can be a claim and a demand: something that must be displayed in specific ways so as to access the privileges of full relational citizenship. But there are other ways in which relational displays can be critical. In conclusion I briefly consider relational displays that are critical *of* family, and how they might be located in a critical-reflexive sociology of display.

In Britain and elsewhere there are histories of endeavours to create alternatives *to* family (Weeks 1991). These were often critical of 'the family' and viewed it as a site of political and personal struggle. They acknowledged that, in addition to practices of love, care and commitment, families could also involve practices of inequality, abuse, exploitation and so on. These endeavours and the criticisms of family that informed them highlight the dangers of assuming that everyone would or should claim family and alert us to the risks of sociologically scripting families in an uncritical way. One interesting question is why displays of relationships that are critical of family tend to be invisible, both in the broader culture and sociologically. Sociologically, we should be sceptical of any essentialist answer to this question that posits the 'natural' importance and resilience of families. Instead, by adapting Plummer's (1995) analysis of personal stories, we can suggest that alternative or critical displays of family are weak displays within our culture because audiences (including sociologists) seem unwilling to receive, interpret and validate them as desirable or viable alternatives to family. A critical-reflexive sociology would ask why our relational imagination is so limited.

There is a risk that in sociologically scripting relational displays *as* family ones we reduce diverse and creative displays of care, love and commitment to family ones. This, in turn, risks making family seem like the most enduring, resilient and 'natural' relationship. In short, by uncritically deploying the family frame to script relational displays we risk making invisible alternative relational realities and possibilities. This shores up family as a privileged relational form, and leaves unchallenged the framing mechanisms that support relational hierarchies and inequalities. Because of this, we should go beyond the sociology of family display and aim for a critical-reflexive sociology of relational displays.

3
Troubling Displays: The Affect of Gender, Sexuality and Class

Jacqui Gabb

I want to engage with Janet Finch's concept of display as an academic lens through which to understand family relationships, focusing on the utility of the concept but also asking questions about what (or who) gets omitted through this analytical paradigm. Finch (2007) suggests that it is not sufficient for families to be done; they must also be seen to be done in order that these sets of practices are afforded cultural meaning. I concur that the concept of display may be a useful addition to the sociological toolkit, but not primarily because it elucidates how family relationships are presented and rendered meaningful – although it certainly does add clarity to understandings of these processes. Instead I think that it is most useful precisely because it brings into sharp relief the determining factors that shape displays and in doing so the people and forms of relating that are omitted when emotions and interactions are not readily recognisable. In this sense its analytical use is as a sensitising concept, highlighting the need for us to be more attuned to those practices and identities that are in different ways troublesome to display.

I am therefore going to focus on different factors that may shape and/or inhibit family displays and the affect of in/visibility. My aim in this is threefold: to explore how external factors impact on what can and cannot be displayed, to examine the effect this has on the qualitative nature of family relationships, and to consider when and why family relationships are displayed and the particular forms these displays may take. To begin, in the first sections of this chapter, I examine some of the determining factors that trouble the concept of displaying families, notably sexuality, gender and class, and the ways that age and generation play a constitutive role in the shaping of family practices. I contend that a focus on display with its incumbent audience reinforces a normalising gaze that legitimises certain displays at the expense of others. This point raises further questions about the research process, returning us to a more methodologically oriented debate. I consider the ways that research affords meaning to certain displays and in so doing renders 'others' effectively meaningless within the public domain.

In later sections I move on to interrogate whether a focus on display can adequately account for the complexity of relational experience; that is to say, can this analytical lens account for the interiority of relationships? This leads me to reflect on the significance of feelings and the affect of personal biographies. In my discussion, I do not seek to contest the utility of the concept of display as a complementary analytical tool that can advance understandings of how family relationships are materialised. However, I do want to draw attention to the problematic of researching private lives which are by definition experienced as personal and which often comprise defended, conflicting and emotionally messy interwoven strands of subjectivity and relationality, the projected meanings of which may be unclear. I want to suggest that we should not only focus on displaying families but should also be mindful of what is happening at the edges and behind the scenes of the narrative on display.

To illustrate my argument I draw on empirical data from two research projects, *Perverting Motherhood?* and *Behind Closed Doors*. These qualitative studies examined experiences and understandings of intimacy and the impact of sexuality on lesbian and heterosexual parent families. *Perverting Motherhood?* was an empirical study of sexuality experiences in lesbian parent households. In-depth, semi-structured interviews were completed with eighteen lesbian mothers and thirteen of their children. Fieldwork was completed over a twelve-month period in 2000 through 2001. The timing of this research is significant, in that data collection took place while Section 28 (1988) was being repealed and before the introduction of Civil Partnership (2004) legislation.[1] The impact of these contextual factors will be addressed within my analysis. *Behind Closed Doors* was an ESRC-funded project (RES-000–22-0854) that used a combination of different qualitative methods to explore experiences and understandings of intimacy and sexuality in families. Fieldwork was completed over a fourteen- month period in 2005–6. Data were collected from ten families in total (nine heterosexual parent households and one lesbian parent household), comprising nine mothers, five fathers and ten children. In both studies there was diversity in family form, socio-economic background, ethnicity and religious belief, although given the sample sizes diversity is inevitably limited and findings cannot be mapped onto wider trends in the population. All families were resident in the North of England in the United Kingdom.

The effect of 'sexual/ity stories' on the display of family

In this first section I want to focus on the effect of 'sexual/ity stories' and how these shape what can and cannot be displayed. In the United Kingdom, most contemporary sociological analyses now feature the foundational ideas of David Morgan who coined the term 'family practices'. The value of this conceptual framework is that it shifts the analytical focus away from determining culturally prescribed forms of family towards diverse sets of interactions that combine to produce families through their 'location in wider systems of meaning' (Morgan 1996: 190). What Finch argues, and the point that I want to unpick, is that *'families need to be "displayed" as well as "done"* in order to register as meaningful in wider culture' (Finch 2007: 66). The contention is that some relationships require demonstrable action if they are to achieve recognisable family status. However, what goes unsaid within this assertion is that the *compulsion to be displayed* can render some individuals and groups without the capacity to be seen. The concept of display may aim to capture the processes through which family relationships are rendered meaningful, but it does so at the expense of invisible others.

The salience of heteronormative models and the impact of cultural norms on displays of family should not be underestimated. In my research on lesbian parent families it was clear that lesbian mothers were crucially aware of the significance of outward facing displays of family and how these shaped and were shaped by everyday relational experience. For lesbians and gay parents, family life tends not to be taken-for-granted and all parties are required to constantly work and rework ideas of family. There may be widespread cultural shifts in ideas and experience of family (Williams 2004) and Civil Partnership legislation does afford parental rights and a degree of legitimacy to lesbian and gay parents in the eyes of the law, but on the ground heteronormative understandings of family are harder to destabilise, so too homophobia. The determining characteristic of parental roles remains 'hetero-gender' (Ingraham 1996), being materialised through female/mother and male/father descriptors that map onto women and men.

Notwithstanding advances in sexual rights, the collapsing together of gender and parenting roles can leave lesbian and gay parents in a precarious position without the discursive tools to display the meaningfulness of their relationships. Language affords meaning to bodies and these 'bodies that matter' (Butler 1993) are displayed through the materiality of language. For example lesbian 'other mothers' (that is to say non-biological mothers) in many ways remain without maternity both on a social level and often in terms of self-perception as well. 'Other mothers' may do the *job of mothering* and may be recognised as a mother when they are doing this role, however this does not necessarily equate with being named as 'mothers' within their families and/or translate into individual identification with the category 'mother'. In my research many 'other mothers' struggled to embrace the identity of mother, believing that *being* a mother was something that was earned over time and/or embodied through maternal labour – at least one of which they did not experience (Gabb 2005a). Their biological separation from childbirth was often accentuated through post-partum mother-child interactions such as breastfeeding and the time spent in early childrearing, time accorded to 'birth mothers' through statutory maternity leave and/or personal decisions to be 'full-time mums'.

> *Janis:*   I wouldn't feel uneasy with it [mother], but it would feel a bit false because I'm not, I'm not physically her mother but also I haven't done .... half the things that would give me the right to have that term if you see what I mean.

Janis and her partner conceived their child as a lesbian couple through donor insemination, and as such they could be seen as the vanguard of lesbian parent family formations. However the 'natural' conjoining of embodied experiences of maternity with understandings of *being* a mother leave Janis (the 'other mother') feeling that she does not have the right to claim this identity. This sentiment was not uncommon and it mirrors perceptions of step-parenthood (Ribbens McCarthy et al. 2003) which suggest that if the embodied category is already filled, then the 'step' or 'other' mother/father can only approximate the original. The sense that the category of mother was already occupied (by the 'birth mother') led several 'other mothers' in my study to queer the heteronormative; to identify themselves more as fathers than mothers. They tended to use this descriptor ironically but it also accurately described their parental role within normatively defined understandings of family – primary wage earner, secondary 'hands off' parent and so on. In this way gender was 'troubled' in everyday family practices, being done and undone in multiple and contradictory ways (Gabb 2005a: 592). Displaying families within this shifting nexus was not, however, an easy task. Lesbian mothers often experienced the invisibility of their role and/or their inability to easily display their family relationships as a source of frustration, annoyance and in some cases a cause of heart-felt distress.

Mothers' difficulty in categorising and naming the 'other mother' was equally experienced by many children. Parents recounted and children spoke about how they at times struggled to fit the messiness of their family forms into the social categories and familial lexicon which is available to them. They just did not have the narrative resources to accurately display their families in the heteronormative contexts they inhabited. Some referred to the 'other mother' as a 'best friend', 'like a dad', or by forename and in some instances a 'second mother', 'like a mum' or simply 'mum'. The cultural meaning ascribed to the relationship that was invoked was simultaneously meaningful and irrelevant. In some cases the terminology used hinted at ambivalence and/or a sense of unease, putting into words feelings that might be ordinarily much harder to articulate. In most cases children perceived their lives as lacking nothing and/or no one. Even in this untroubled scenario, however, problems were encountered in displaying family. Children often needed to be highly skilled in the arts of concealment and disclosure, with feelings of anxiety often centring on their experiences in school.

Schools have been the setting for fraught political battles on the legitimacy of lesbian and gay sexuality. In the United Kingdom, Section 28 may have been removed from the statute books and, even during its existence, in practice many schools paid little heed to the edicts that were enshrined in this homophobic legislation. But the tolerance of individual teachers and good intentions of some school governing boards do not prohibit bullying in the playground. In these spaces children (especially teenagers) were often highly circumspect about who to confide in and when such confidences were safe. Many children in my study spoke of their pride in their families and personally had no problems with their mothers' sexuality, but they nevertheless felt uncomfortable in displaying their families among a peer audience. Younger children were typically less cautious and many openly described their families as having two mothers but whether these disclosures became more candid as they entered the challenging territory of adolescence and the high school playground I do not know. As children conceived in the context of lesbian and gay civil partnerships pass through the educational system, it remains to be seen whether displaying families in all their diverse forms gets easier and/or the audience becomes any more receptive. The depressing regularity of brutal and sometimes fatal homophobic attacks on gay men in particular suggests that the impact of Civil Partnership legislation and professed advances in social tolerance of lesbian and gay male sexuality are often hard to perceive. Public spaces tend to remain sites of high risk for those who display their homosexuality, especially for young men.

Even when parents felt personally at ease with their role and identity and were secure in their belief that their displays of family demonstrated the closeness of these relationships, the *reception* and *comprehension* of these displays could not be guaranteed. Physical hostility was rare but verbal abuse and embodied admonishments were experienced at some point by most families. I concur with Finch when she talks about the significance of *recognition* (Finch 2007: 74) but not all recognisable displays receive affirming receptions. While it is true to say that if relationships are perceived as family and they resemble those of family then they are family. For lesbian parents and their families, however, there is also a degree of *misrecognition* that frequently occurs; a practice that serves to undermine the legitimacy of these relationships. Signs of lesbian sexuality that may connote lesbian-ness and which may be identifiable in certain contexts such as the nightclub or gay bar, can be obscured by the presence of a child (Gabb 2005b). While cultural shifts have increased social tolerance of certain forms of lesbian and gay 'coupling', the overriding effect of normative discourses tie mothers and children to the heterosexual reproductive narrative, obscuring all other readings and rendering the display of lesbian parenthood invisible. Though some lesbian mothers may perceive their families to be 'obvious' or unmistakable, those outside 'queer culture' can remain oblivious because they do not know how to *read* the display.

> *Matilda:*   A lot, I mean people have said that to us quite a lot, like at the doctor's surgery when, you know, antenatal and that, I think even maybe at the hospital, they do assume we're sisters and they think we look alike [... .] because that's the only way they can interpret it or that's the immediate way they interpret it and that kind of sort of ease ... .

In accounts of lesbian motherhood, many of the women spoke to me about being mistaken for sisters. This misrecognition is interesting on several fronts. It acknowledges the intimacy of the two women and their familial proximity both to each other and to the child. Notwithstanding the closeness of this affinity, the 'coupling' however cannot be put into words that *fit* the display which is on offer. Civil partnerships and the increasing number of women who are conceiving children as a female couple have raised public awareness of lesbian parenting, but cultural norms remain stubbornly attached. The 'natural' conjunction of mother-child often displaces all other readings. For two women to be *this close* they must be related and therefore they must be siblings. To reinforce this belief, and despite visual evidence to the contrary, familial embodied likeness is often found where none actually exists.

Theorising on the 'transformation of intimacy' (Giddens 1992) and the material effects of greater individualisation on the relationships that are valued and maintained (Bauman 2003; Beck and Beck-Gersheim 1995) suggests that we live in a time of sexual fluidity that is characterised by degrees of choice and which may herald a kaleidoscopic display of relational forms. For many individuals, however, there remain strong attachments to normative ideas of 'family' (Ribbens McCarthy et al. 2003) which leave those living in-between sexual and familial spaces feeling 'out of place' in most scenarios (Gabb 2005a). While Finch may cite research on families of choice

(Weeks et al. 2001) as a good example of how 'family-like' relationships are authenticated through their semblance to wider cultural norms, the shift from queer-sexual identities to recognisably meaningful and legitimised familial ways of living is not always an easy transition. Moreover, holding up 'families of choice' as an analytical and experiential exemplar of displaying families in action disregards the fact that this grouping has been effectively unpicked for glossing over as it does the individual tensions that are experienced (Gabb 2004b; Gross 2005). This is not to say that I concur with dismissive critiques of valuable and insightful research in this vein. 'Families of choice' literature is not uniform nor does it hinge on social privilege which bestows the option to choose. But it is fair to say that some formative work in this area has been inclined to leave to one side those who do not feel 'at home' in this community-oriented versioning of intimacy and/or who, for *personal* reasons, struggle to fit comfortably within this 'scenic' view.

My focus so far in this chapter has been on lesbian and gay parent families. It is not, however, only same-sex parents who have to develop strategies to manage troublesome sexuality. In families, constant boundary management of sexuality of all persuasions is required in order to offset 'risks' and/or unruly manifestations of any kind. Across both datasets, it was evident that there were many factors which affected how parents negotiate sexuality at home including personal biography, cultural context, age and generation. Social policies, legislation and prevailing ideas on codes of conduct also undoubtedly have a significant impact. One further factor which often receives far less serious attention is the material effects of sexual/ity stories which circulate through the media, especially those which report high profile cases – such as tragic instances of child abuse and/or those associated with 'celebrities' (Gabb 2008). For example, one mother from the *Behind Closed Doors* study recounted a 'media story' which she said had irrevocably changed the ways that she and her husband experience and display parent-child intimacy.

In 1996 the partner of Julia Somerville (a former BBC newsreader) walked into a local chemist and handed over a roll of exposed film containing what he perceived to be innocent family snapshots. On processing the film, an employee became 'suspicious' about several bath-time pictures which depicted the naked bodies of father and child and the employee handed over the photographs to the police for investigation. Despite quickly finding there was no case to answer, the story was somehow 'leaked' to the press and as a consequence was widely discussed on television and in the papers and for a while became a focused topic of conversation among the general public.

This whole sequence of events must have been personally distressing for the Somerville family and it has been subsequently roundly criticised in many quarters. The creation and circulation of child pornography is certainly not a trivial matter and the police were duty bound to look into the case; as such they only followed due process. But the cultural significance of the allegations and the *impact* of this kind of 'story' on ordinary families' intimate practices have not been generally acknowledged. Notwithstanding the adjudged innocence of the pictures, the media hyperbole and concomitant public discussion on the legitimacy of displaying such parent-child activities rendered *the experience* itself a source of potential risk. As a result of this 'story', the mother and father in my study spoke about needing to be 'very careful' about what displays they make public. They have revised their code of conduct and set clear-cut age boundaries around parent-child interactions. While both parents believed the 'story' to be 'ridiculous', it has nevertheless changed their practice and display of family relationships.

The strength of these parents' reaction can in part be attributed to a combination of personal circumstances. The mother is British Asian and lives in a small town with a predominantly white U.K. population. She therefore perceives that her racial origin makes her family highly visible in the local community, a factor that increased the level of her anxiety and, as a consequence, the degree to which this family's display of intimate behaviour was adjusted. Furthermore both parents work in health and child welfare professions and their re-actions were in part attributed to their 'insider' status. Knowing what they did, they were particularly cognisant of the potential for misreadings and/or false allegations around father-child intimacy and they therefore felt that they needed to be above 'suspicion'.

Concerns and awareness of this kind were expressed by other parents with similar professional lives and also by many lesbian parents who perceived their families to be subject to far greater scrutiny by virtue of their sexuality. However, the single most significant factor which instigated changes in the patterning of affective behaviour in families was gender. In Western culture father-child intimacy is now generally encouraged but paradoxically the innocence of such activities is seldom taken-for-granted. Male sexuality remains typically characterised as predatory (Gabb 2004a); fathers are, first and foremost, men and, as such, fatherhood is risky *by default*. Mothers spoke about policing adult male-child interactions 'just in case', restricting embodied contact to immediate family and generally erring on the side of caution. Fathers talked of their frustrations and concerns in having to be always mindful of how their actions might be perceived (See also Doucet, Chapter 5).

Gender and class: the silencing of affect

The significance of gender in the dynamic of intimate family life cannot be understated and surfaces in many ways. Traditionally, understandings of the gendered patterning of family living have tended to be centred on women as 'wives' and mothers. Recently, popular and political attention has shifted towards fathers and the role, responsibilities and meanings of fatherhood. Research has begun to trace these changing attitudes towards men and fatherhood; work that is characterised by a focus on the significance/insignificance of gender (Dermott 2008; Doucet 2006a; Featherstone 2009). Studies differ in their interpretations of what is shaping shifts in practices and cultural imaginations of fatherhood, but leaving to one side these points of contestation and the obdurate inequalities that characterise gendered domestic roles and responsibilities, there is agreement on underlying differences between the ways that men and women *do* parenting including how they display their feelings.

In data from the *Behind Closed Doors* study, gender differences were marked. Women tended to be far more eloquent than men in their descriptions of their emotions. This is not surprising given that many of these women had previously worked through their feelings and/or rehearsed 'emotion stories' in conversations with female family and friends. They were more practiced and thus readily able to display an affective account of themselves. Notwithstanding such differences, we should be wary of promoting the cultural versioning of gender scripts which tell of men's emotional ineptitude. The presupposition that men do not really 'do' emotions and that gender can be mapped onto affective behaviour may do a disservice to both men and women (Gabb 2008).

In the *Behind Closed Doors* project one mother traced gendered practices of intimacy across her life. Describing her childhood she said that her mother was always very easy to hug; in contrast, expressions of affection between her and her father were 'difficult', especially as she started to 'grow up' and 'got too big' for such displays. This was a recurrent story across the dataset. Fathers were often extremely self-conscious about openly displaying family relationships with children who were becoming young adults. As men they felt uncomfortable with holding hands or embracing a pubescent offspring. Fathers did not, however, totally withdraw from their relationships; instead many started to show affection in less tactile ways. In one family the father began doing things for his daughter such as making fitted wardrobes, practices that were designed to demonstrate the enduring closeness of the father-daughter relationship.

Notwithstanding men's struggle to express their emotions, there was no sense that they were any less feeling. Instead, close analysis of data demonstrated that fathers often *displayed* emotions in ways that were not readily understood and/or recognisable as affection – the building of wardrobes being one case in point! In some instances intimate exchanges between father and child were ostensibly indiscernible to those outside the family; invisible to those who do not know their encoded registers of emotion. In another case, Jeff (a young single parent) talked about how his father had never been 'lovey-dovey' but that he knows 'me dad love me to bits ... it's intuition ... he's saying it indirectly'. When asked how he expresses his love for his father he replied:

> *Jeff:* At Christmas I got me dad something he wanted and it was more expensive than what me mam got, but I got me mam what she wanted as well ... and me dad got some tools. I think me dad realises how much I spend on him, he knows, he's not daft me dad, he knows how much I spend and if I spend a bit more I think he knows, in a way, that's my way of saying 'Thanks, you've been brilliant' ...

Jeff grew up in a family where money was always in short supply. His emotional and financial investment in the exchange of gifts as a codified means to demonstrate affection could thus be attributed both to his (male) exclusion from the feminine-defined cultural repertoires of love and emotional disclosure and also to his economically deprived family background. 'Making something from nothing' remains a source of pride for Jeff; displaying depth of feeling through the emotional investment of time in creating home-cooked meals, enjoying 'cheap' days out and simply *being* together as family. Spending a bit more money on his dad at Christmas is therefore extremely significant and meaningful. In this scenario Jeff, like many men who took part in the study and other male relatives who were described by participants, tended not to use words or gestures that were easily decipherable. It was only through the recursive design of the fieldwork, returning again and again to families and using different methods to approach different aspects of family relationship, that men's emotional vocabulary fully came to light.

As these complex narratives unfolded it became evident that particular encoded displays of emotion and family relationships could be identified among working-class families. Taking account of these working-class emotion currencies is crucial. Research has shown how understandings of 'good parenthood' are often filtered through class assumptions (Armstrong 2006). Determining ideas of 'bad mothering' are fixed onto perceived practices of working-class parenthood, making working-class mothers marginalised, disrespected and blamed for many social problems associated with unruly and/or unhealthy childhood and youth (Gillies 2006). Perceptions and experiences of parenthood are shaped by class positioning, educational advantage and cultural capital, intersecting factors that are compounded by the illegitimacy of lesbian and gay sexuality (Taylor 2009).

Focusing on the materiality of class, Les Back (2007) has commented on the ways that working-class cultures are embodied in certain practices of intimacy but that these displays of relating and emotional investment often go unnoticed. For example Back examines how particular forms of tattooing are synonymous with working-class culture, such as having the names of partners and children or the insignia of a beloved football club proudly displayed upon the skin. He claims that such signs of allegiance and devotion often fall beneath the sociological radar because these forms of communication and displays of affection do not fit with middle-class frameworks of meaning that increasingly rely on articulations of emotions, epitomised by the compulsion to disclose our every feeling (Giddens

1992). Working-class 'inscriptions of love' are carved into their 'fleshy canvas' using registers of feeling which typically go unspoken.

> Love is given a name: it is incarnate. But this commitment is not made in elaborated speeches. It is performed rather than described. It is a kind of illocutionary love, a love that is expressed without painstaking announcement. (Back 2007: 82)

For Back, the task is not only to acknowledge the existence of these 'alternative modalities of love' but to *expand the sociological imagination* so that we become attuned to these silent and silenced voices. Working-class lives are often characterised as expressionless, lacking in both sensitivity and commitment; Back reminds us that this is not the case. There is not a lack of emotional capacity, it is academics and social commentators who need to develop our *research capacity*. We need to employ a broader spectrum of senses: to listen and hear, to see and notice; to take account of the wide-ranging registers of feeling that are in operation. Returning to the stories that emerged during the course of my research I have uncovered so many of these invisible modalities of love. In many ways these span across the social spectrum. For example, in one family a middle-class mother repeatedly mentioned 'cup of tea and a chat'. This affective shorthand symbolised her attempts to make connections with various members of her family. It was her gift of intimacy; without florid expression or exuberant demonstration it was her way of displaying her love. In this and other circumstances a cup of tea does important, often unrecognised emotional labour (Dorrer et al. 2008; Punch et al. 2009).

I do however agree with Back (2007) in that focusing the analytical gaze on these wordless modalities is particularly helpful in taking account of those who are pushed to the edges of dominant mainstream culture. Returning to Jeff, mentioned previously, his expression of gratitude and love for his father through his more generous Christmas gift, demonstrates the need to examine emotional displays beyond normative models; to stretch the conceptual imagination. From the outside it would be all too easy to read the intimate relationship between Jeff and his father as affection free. They do not say 'I love you' and there is nothing to suggest that physical expressions of intimacy are the norm, in fact the opposite. Their relational interactions remain unreadable and therefore potentially misunderstood by those beyond immediate family, or indeed beyond Jeff and his father. This raises several crucial questions for Finch's concept of 'displaying families'. Are such relationships as these, which are not readily apparent, any less socially meaningful just because we – the audience – cannot recognise them as significant? In 'translating' individual displays, can we ever coherently account for the interiority of emotions? Finch suggests that *all* relationships require an element of display to sustain them as family relationships. In the next sections I want to unpick these points, interrogating how we, as family researchers, need to refine our analytical art in order to make sense of the multilayered visible and invisible displays that are portrayed.

Making sense of displays: the significance of methods

To begin, I want to unravel Jeff's relational 'story', and how this emerged through the research process, through the combination of qualitative mixed methods. In the *Behind Closed Doors* study there were often notable differences amongst data generated in different methods. This is perhaps unsurprising given that different methods were designed to elicit data on different aspects of family living (Gabb 2009). Emotion maps located *where* intimate encounters occurred in different spaces around the home. Diaries produced data on *when* intimacy happened and showed *how* participants conceptually and narratively framed these emotion exchanges. Biographical narrative interviews elicited reflective accounts that spanned across participants' life course. Vignettes, photo interviews and focus group discussion of third-party scenarios garnered data on a social level, focusing attention on the cultural frameworks that shaped participants' opinions. Pieced together, mixed methods data illustrated the patterning of family practice and emotions across generations; the building of subjectivity through past and present experiences. The impact of these contextual factors on events and experiences across the life course cannot be underestimated.

For example, in describing his relationship with his father, his account was full of emotional awkwardness. In contrast, when speaking *as* a father, Jeff's descriptions of his relationship with his own children demonstrated great emotional fluency:

> *Jeff (diary):*   M&M are very happy this morning because we are going to see Grandma and Granddad had lots of kisses & cuddles for them. Had lots of fun and laughs. Had macaroni cheese for tea (that's the kids' favourite meal). Molly went to bed give me kisses & cuddles for me and so did Mike ...

Jeff used his research diary to display the *quality* of his family life and the closeness of the father-children relationship. Here, and elsewhere, he recounted his pride in being recently awarded the custody of his children from the mother through the courts. During this protracted judicial process he had to 'prove' his parenting capabilities to a wider *public* audience. It is therefore not surprising that he was extremely eloquent in his descriptions of parent-child affection and invested so deeply in the idea of family. Jeff attends classes in parenting skills at his local Children's Centre and is *actively* crafting sets of practices and relationships with the 'assistance' of health, child welfare and family support agencies which advocate a particular and recognisable model of 'good parenting'. In this way his *display of family* says more about the current *ideal of family* than it does about the emotional connections that are experienced in their everyday relational context. This does not question in any way the integrity of Jeff's parenting or his genuine depth of feeling for his children. Instead, it foregrounds context and the personal motivations that may impact on encoded displays of family, sensitising us to individual circumstances.

The idea of displaying families is particularly useful in this regard because it requires us to take account of the complexities and multi-dimensional factors that shape the display of relationships. It encourages us to drill down through what is *on display*, to consider how different circumstances affect family practices. The perceived need to *be seen to be doing family,* that comes to the fore in particular moments, is a characteristic that can be found in many studies of family living, as people perform family for a wider audience. Finch cites two examples; the first is step-parent families and how fathers in these circumstances (or moments) may be compelled to display their parenting so that it still counts even though their everyday familial role may have lessened. The second example refers to how the patterning of relationships necessarily 'evolves' as children grow up and loosen connections with their parents. She suggests that, in these contexts, processes of relating need to be displayed to re-establish and/or consolidate attachments as 'family relationships which work' (Finch 2007: 72). My analysis of the affect of sex/uality stories and the impact of gender, generation and class all support Finch's assertion on the significance of particular moments of display.

The *recognition* of family relationships 'which work' does, however, presupposes that their effectiveness is achieved, at least in part, through their successful externalisation. In this sense the concept of displaying families is somewhat problematic, in that it could unintentionally denigrate the *emotional value of relational experience*. For those on the margins, saying that experience alone is insufficient to produce meaning, it adds a further layer of social exclusion. For some, experience may be the only legitimising factor in their relationships. On this point I therefore disagree with Finch, who argues that:

> There is a real sense in which relationships do not exist as *family* relationships unless they can be displayed successfully. They cannot exist solely in my own consciousness. They need to be understood and accepted as such by others. (Finch 2007: 79)

My contention with this assertion stems from two intersecting factors. First, the argument imposes a normalising gaze through which we measure 'successfulness', both of the relationships that are on display and the legitimacy of these relationships as family. This assertion starts from the centre ground where there is a presumption of shared understanding around 'what is family', 'what is family-like' and the corollary 'what is *not* family'. I have shown that by starting from the margins – where cultural scripts are often fractured and contested – we can begin to see the diverse ways that family narratives and relationships are being done, redone and undone *without recognisable displays*. In these scenarios family practices are taking place but displays may fall outside the registers of cultural intelligibility and therefore what is *on display* may bear little semblance to family scripts. Second, the existence of relationships is not wholly reliant on public-facing performances to make them meaningful (that is to say recognisable as family). Unseen relationships and family practices which are invisible to anyone beyond those *doing* the relating can be meaningful and personally enhancing for those involved. It is this latter point that I want to address in the final and concluding section of this chapter, focusing attention on the in/significance of audience and researching the un-displayed.

The complexity of emotions: researching what is un-displayed

Finch acknowledges that understandings of 'my family' are personal and remain 'deeply rooted in individual biographies' (Finch 2007: 66) but paradoxically the impact of these personal lives on the displays that may be enacted is not taken up. There is attention to the fluidity of families and how different relationships are 'continually evolving' (Finch 2007: 69). This acknowledges how relationships may be shaped over the course of time through intersecting personal, social and historical circumstances but it does not however account for the significance of feelings and life stories and how these affect the personal narratives that are experienced and which may be put on display. I want to now think about the affect of personal biographies with reference to recent advances in understanding offered through psycho-social approaches to studies of intimate relationships.

The development of U.K. family sociology has followed an interesting course. Emerging from its functionalist past where gendered patterns of parenting were seen to 'marry up' with the needs of the socio-economic family unit, contemporary research now focuses on how relationships are made and remade through everyday 'family practices' which gain cultural meaning through the significance afforded to these practices (Morgan 1996). In this sense the idea of displaying families does add clarity to how we understand what constitutes family, as constellations of adults and children only *become* families when they are recognised as such (Finch 2007). But in some ways it also serves to obscure other dimensions, that is, how individuals, or for that matter certain groups of individuals, *personally experience* family relationships.

There is an identifiable psycho-social shift that is occurring in some areas of family studies which is concerned with intersections between the biographical, social and emotional factors that shape relationships

(Gabb 2008). Much of this work is reliant on determining psychoanalytic explanations that theoretically interpret emotions and behaviour. Leaving this body of work to one side, I do believe that sociologically informed psycho-social analyses can equally make sense of personal lives and the multi-dimensional complexity of family living. The concept of displaying families does not prohibit taking account of the interiority of relational practices, but neither does it situate this individualised component at the analytical heart. In studying lesbian lives I have become increasingly aware of how experiences and understandings are not shaped by women's sexuality per se. but by a combination of personal circumstances including class, race, biography and current context. Together these experiences shape lesbian parenthood, being *structured through feeling*.

Emotions are seldom straightforward and for many lesbians, becoming a parent is a fraught and individually troublesome path. Uncertainties may derive from a multitude of social-personal factors which span the life course; the impact of heteronormative culture often increases and/or compounds underlying feelings of insecurity. Psycho-social research recognises these feelings of self doubt, anger, ambivalence and insecurity as part of ordinary registers of emotion (Roseneil 2007). The fact that society automatically recognises a mother, father and child as a family leaves those outside this framework to scrabble around the edges to claim personal meaning. Being recognised as family is undoubtedly affirming, but being recognised as *like a family* or *family-like* is certainly not the same thing. Lesbian parents feel this exclusionary difference – it has a meaningful and largely negative affect. 'Performances' of identity (or family) may evidence the artificiality of the original (Butler 1990) but for parents this 'educational' role can be sometimes perceived as a burden. Thinking about whether it is personally safe to hold hands and/or the impact this may have upon your child is emotionally consequential both to the individuals involved and to the forms of family that can be displayed. The concept of display must always take account of these emotional stories and how they impact on what can and cannot be displayed.

The affect of gender is similarly influential. In the *Behind Closed Doors* project, most men spoke about wanting to attain positive father-child relationships. Some actively reconstructed fatherhood around a feminine-defined model, being demonstrably affectionate with their children and valuing 'disclosing intimacy' (Jamieson 1998). These fathers' desire to achieve and/or *be seen to achieve* increased parent-child contact and emotional connection may be due to a variety of factors. They could be a response to social pressures which advocate greater paternal involvement; a consequence of wider changes and the loosening of categorical masculine-feminine roles; or they may be shaped through particular sets of *personal* circumstances. It is often the *combination* of these social-biographical factors which impact on men's capacity to display the interiority of families. For many men their emotions and relational worlds can all too easily fail to register on both cultural and analytical radars. If we are to fully understand the shifting registers of experience, patterns of intimacy and meanings of family, then we need to find strategies to engage with the wide-ranging, encoded and/or *un-displayed* actions and words which are affectively telling. To decipher these emotional tales requires detailed and careful analysis of participants' complex, guarded and often conflicting data.

For example, Jeff, the single father cited previously, is highly practiced in his display of family. He skilfully crafts past and present narratives of kin in his diary and elsewhere in his oral descriptions of childhood and family events. But these meaningful *social stories* conceal other underlying emotional stories of self and relationality. Embedded in Jeff's data were threads of pain, distress, ambivalence and anger, *negative emotions* that were never openly acknowledged or discussed. On the surface and on a practical level, Jeff is a most resilient young man who is succeeding to raise two young children on his own, against the odds. His achievements are significant. What 'joined up' analysis of qualitative mixed methods data added to understandings of his story, was the constant work that this required.

I want to suggest that where ideas of display could prove to be a particularly useful addition to the analytical toolkit is in focusing attention on *what* is being displayed in order to generate understanding of *why* these displays appear in the forms that they do. In this way *what is not displayed* moves into the research frame and questions about the constitutive elements of people's emotional stories begin to be answered through their personal narrations of self. The concept of 'displaying families' can add another dimension to studies of family relationships, but it does so *indirectly*, reminding us that we need to be cognisant of the *invisible* displays of families that we encounter in the field. Its value is that it prompts us to develop research capacity that is attentive to the diverse 'narratives' which do not fit recognisable displays of families. I contend that this expansion of the sociological imagination is crucial; otherwise we perpetuate normalising discourses which privilege certain sets of attachments and forms of relationships and erase the value of others which do not have readily available scripts and/or that are already demonised by sets of moral values which determine what displays affectively count. I agree with Finch (2007: 78): By focusing on the ways that people display their family relationships we can begin to capture the extending repertoire of relating practices which people draw on to show they care for one another. As family researchers we are still learning, developing and refining the conceptual frameworks and research tools that we use; a process that can only enhance understandings of multi-dimensional displays of family that are presented in all their myriad formations.

Note

1. Section 28 of the British Local Government Act (May 1988) prohibited local authorities from 'intentionally promot[ing] homosexuality' and 'pretended family relationships' within schools. It was repealed in Scotland in June 2000 and in the rest of the United Kingdom by Section 122 of the Local Government Act in November 2003. The Civil Partnership Act (2004) afforded lesbians and gay men almost equal rights to those acquired through heterosexual marriage. Rights included equitable treatment for financial matters, such as inheritance, pensions provision and life insurance. Under Section 72 of the Act, civil partners were afforded 'parental responsibilities' for children, equal to those of other stepparents. Partners were able to apply for residence or contact orders and for the financial provision (ordinarily in the form of maintenance) for any children. Adoption provisions were also amended to treat civil partners the same as married couples.

Part II
Applying the Concept

4
Displaying Motherhood: Representations, Visual Methods and the Materiality of Maternal Practice

Mary Jane Kehily and Rachel Thomson

Introduction

In her 2007 paper 'Displaying Families' Janet Finch argues for the need to develop Morgan's notion of family practices to include an awareness of the ways in which families must engage in display in order to negotiate the distanciation of the family over time and space, and the recognition of the validity of these practices. For the family to have 'social reality', to be recognised as a family (2007: 74), she argues, it may be necessary to perform specific practices and to have these acknowledged. Although the gaining of recognition may be felt most acutely by families who are in some ways marginalised, the demand to display family practices is common to all families, although the intensity of such practices may vary over time. Although Finch employs the term 'display' she does not intend to focus simply on embodied or visual practices, but includes family narratives and naming practices in her definition of the tools of display. However, her account does not engage explicitly with the wider landscape of cultural and visual representations of the family. For Finch the concept of 'display' is used to encourage us to think about the audience, reception and recognition of family practices, consistent with the sociological framing of stories outlined by Plummer (1995), which not only includes the conditions for a story to be articulated, but also the existence of an audience and their willingness to hear and recognise a story. Yet the notion of 'display' also brings with it the potential to connect family practices to wider landscapes of representation – those imagined families that circulate within popular culture and which incite and discipline our desires, ideas and practices (Smart 2007). Moreover, it may be that in particular moments the visual and the embodied become heightened elements of personal experience and governance. Imogen Tyler (2001) for example, convincingly documents a shift to the 'spectacular' in representations of contemporary pregnancy, with previous notions of confinement displaced by the imperative to display the pregnant body. The development of new technologies for representation also transform what it is possible to display with infertility treatments, ultrasound and three-dimensional images of the foetus extending and disrupting notions of intimacy and the public.

In this chapter we focus on one of those moments within the life course that is associated with what Finch characterises as an 'intensification' of display. Conception and the public recognition of pregnancy demand a redrawing of the boundaries of the self and of intimacy – initially through narratives (Thomson and Kehily 2009) and increasingly through consumption and the display and recognition of the pregnant body. These practices of display do not take place within a neutral environment. Rather, pregnancy is framed within a broad common culture of motherhood that is both highly visual and intensely narrated and populated by a proliferation of objects, equipment and expert and consumer advice (Baraitser 2008; Clarke 2004; Hardyment 2007; Martens 2009). In order to research pregnancy and birth within contemporary times it is impossible to abstract narratives and performances from the wider cultural landscape within which representations of mothering abound. Our approach in this chapter demonstrates both our attempts to harness these popular cultural resources as research tools and our interest in the ways in which women experience pregnancy through practices of consumption, display and recognition. We aim to contribute to the concept of displaying families by illustrating the ways in which first-time mothers-to-be may be implicated in modes of display that constitute the emergence of 'family'. Our analysis suggests that the material and representational domains of motherhood have a significant impact upon women's identities as mothers-to-be and on their developing awareness of what it means to be a mother in contemporary times, and thus on the kinds of display practices that they themselves engaged in. In preparing for the birth of their first child, women embark upon a maternal project that creates a 'new' family marked by engagements with the realms of consumption and representation that can be seen as incitements to display.

Methodology

This chapter draws upon data gathered during the course of a project funded by the Economic and Social Research Council: The Making of Modern Motherhoods: Memories, Identities, Representations.[1] The study explores motherhood as a changing social identity by looking *across* the experiences of first-time mothers, mapping similarities and differences against practices of solidarity and distinction. We also look *back* through the accounts of their mothers and grandmothers in order to ask how identities are negotiated intergenerationally within the intimacy of family life. Within the context of social change marked by women's increased participation in education and the labour force, we document moments of intergenerational rupture and change within families triggered by the arrival of a new generation. The social polarisation of motherhood is one of the most distinctive demographic trends of the post-war period, reflected in a movement towards late motherhood for the majority and early motherhood for a minority. In the contemporary era, motherhood is an arena in which socio-economic differences among women are defined and compounded by distinct cultures of childrearing (Byrne 2006; Clarke 2004; Tyler 2008). Within this context we ask: How do women imagine and practise motherhood? What resources and advice do they draw upon (cultural texts, people, products, community)? And how does this fit with other identities?

The chapter is drawn from a data set of sixty-two interviews with first-time mothers and twelve intergenerational case studies. An analysis of popular representations of contemporary mothering was undertaken in parallel with the interview study. Popular resources were identified in an initial questionnaire and integrated into the interview schedule. We also carried out an analysis of magazines aimed at new mothers during the period September 2004 to April 2006. Using digital cameras, visual data gathering methods were used in interviews to document the ways in which first-time mothers prepared for the births of their babies. In this chapter we draw upon those aspects of the research where motherhood is visibly displayed through engagement with representations, material objects/goods and the creation of physical space for the new baby. We consider the place of cultural texts and commodities in mothering practices including engagement with magazines, websites, leaflets, commodities, television, advertising and popular cultural representations of motherhood. Our focus upon the visual and material aspects of the study comments upon the significance of *display* as a site for the unfolding practice of motherhood, the shaping of maternal identities and family relationships. Our approach in this research involved a combination of cultural and sociological analyses and we consciously drew upon popular imagery as a tool for the generation of talk in interviews, as well as for making visual documents of the ways in which women were materialising the impending arrival of a child. This chapter explores and documents three ways in which motherhood is displayed across the project: in visual prompt material integrated into interviews; through analysis of pregnancy magazines; and finally the visual record of women's preparation for birth. We discuss each of these in turn in separate sections, beginning with a framing section on the 'common culture' of mothering to introduce the key themes. Our approach to the ways in which motherhood is displayed does not draw a distinction between methodological enquiry and analytic findings; rather, we draw both together as a way of exploring the enactment of motherhood across the research process as a whole.

The 'common culture' of mothering

The notion of a 'common culture' of youth was developed by Paul Willis and colleagues (1990) to capture the very different ways that young people may be positioned in relation to a shared set of cultural resources. We suggest that a parallel argument can be made in relation to motherhood. We characterise the material and representational dimensions of motherhood as part of the 'common culture' (Willis et al. 1990) of mothering – the routine and everyday existence of mass produced and culturally available representations and commodities that create versions of the maternal in the public sphere. These cultural products become *resources* for new mothers that can be drawn upon to imagine and personalise the project of motherhood. Our study points to some of the ways in which the common culture of mothering is temporally structured and culturally specific. The very idea of imagining motherhood assumes agency, and where women's pregnancies were unplanned or unwanted they struggled to formulate narratives that articulated the kind of mother they would be. Those women who constructed motherhood as part of an explicit project of self tended to have highly developed narratives, drawing (often ironically) on popular cultural resources which in turn construct choice through a series of binary divides between natural and medical births (associated with a commitment to NCT or NHS ante-natal classes); child- and adult-centred parenting (exemplified by the *Baby Whisperer* vs. Gina Ford's *Contented Baby*) and the provision of factual information and lifestyle advice (Hardyment 2007). Although women of all ages and backgrounds drew strategically on the 'common culture' of mothering, it was women in the 26- to 35-years age group who tended to position themselves in relation to these distinctions.

Most of the women we interviewed enjoyed preparing for the arrival of the baby through shopping, sorting and decorating (Young 2005). Our visual data reflect the contrasting situations from which women embarked on this project: some having just a corner of a room or a drawer in which to create a new world, others expanding the project into newly acquired, four-bedroom houses. A minority refused to engage in such activity due to superstition and fear. Material objects were bought, borrowed and received, and the intensive transaction of goods in the final weeks of pregnancy can be seen as mapping the web of obligations that frames the arrival of a new generation. The traffic in commodities within the extended family points to one of the ways in which familial relations may be sustained and nurtured during periods of transition and change. 'Doing' family through gift giving celebrates the arrival of the new baby and simultaneously offers a way of displaying a reconfigured intergenerational line-up in which daughters become mothers and mothers become grandmothers. In keeping with cultural studies and approaches to popular culture we suggest that the publically available 'stuff' of motherhood can be see as part of a 'circuit of cultural production' (du Gay 1997; Hall 1980) in which messages relating to the maternal are encoded by and through media forms. Through engagement with popular culture, women decode these messages and interpret them in diverse ways that make sense within the context of their own lives. The circle joins in the final field of interaction and dialogue in which the myriad interpretations produced by the audience feed into and inform the ways in which further messages are encoded.

Visual prompt material

Our first approach to tracing the ways in which motherhood is displayed lies in the visual prompt material we integrated into the interview schedule for first-time mothers. In this phase of the project we were interested in asking women in the final stages of their first pregnancy to reflect on motherhood both as a personal experience and beyond the immediacy of their personal experience. We selected a range of images from a diverse body of popular cultural sources to facilitate this dialogue. The images of celebrities and comic characters were readily recognisable to women in the U.K. context as high profile figures whose lifestyles saturated popular media forms. Our key aim was to offer women an invitation to explore the boundaries of the common culture of mothering, identifying points of identification and difference by speaking to feelings generated by the images. Our selection of approximately twenty images included advertisements, magazine and newspaper features and promotional material. In most interviews the images were introduced towards the end of the interview and women were asked to comment freely on what they saw. Many of the images highlighted the idea of pregnancy as a time of increased visibility, when women are *on show*. Fashion features encouraged women to indulge in maternity wear to profile the gloriousness of the pregnant tummy. Celebrity pregnancies profiled how to do it or not do it. A feature drawn from a pregnancy magazine entitled *Pregnant and Fabulous* showcased glossy photographs of pregnant celebrities taken as they go to the Oscars, fashion house parties and premiere nights. Wearing designer garments such as an 'off-the-shoulder black dress showing plenty of cleavage', a maroon and gold sari and a red ball gown, celebrities agree that 'you feel more feminine when you're pregnant, sexier'.

One of the celebrities, however, appeared to cross the line, taking pregnant sexiness into more controversial territory. Glamour model and reality TV star Jordan is pictured in the final weeks of pregnancy wearing a cropped, see-through top and size 6 jeans, leaving the bulging tummy fully exposed between the micro garments. While most of our respondents enjoyed the pregnant-and-stunning look modelled so beguilingly by the celebs, they were keen to distance themselves from Jordan's style. 'Improper', 'tarty' and 'ridiculous' sum up many of the responses which comment more broadly on her borderline respectability as a celebrity and a mother-to-be. The invocation of notions of propriety and respectability became recognisable themes in many women's responses to these images, indicating the need to position themselves in relation to these discourses that have an impact upon feminine subjectivity in a general sense (Skeggs 2004) and appear to find renewed focus in pregnancy. We found that women made significant investments in the embodied display of pregnancy, feeling strongly that how you wear your bump matters. Images of pregnant celebrities appear to encode a particular feminine aesthetic, a notion of 'pregnant beauty' (Tyler 2001) that can be both inspirational and regulatory in its appeal to women to measure themselves up against their celebrity counterparts and to compare celebrities with each other.

Two further images arousing strongly felt responses were a photograph of the Marc Jacobs' sculpture of disabled artist Alison Lapper and a photograph of the *Little Britain* character Vicky Pollard. The consensus view on Alison Lapper heralded her as a brave and heroic figure, an 'amazing' women and a mother. By contrast the image of Vicky Pollard produced immediate peals of laughter and derision. As an instantly recognisable parody of young motherhood, the image generated expressions of humour and disgust. The aggressive, shoplifting, pram-face girl in the maelstrom of a troubled life has become associated with excessive working class femininity and particularly 'Chav' identity (Nayak 2006; Tyler 2008), a ubiquitous signifier for the unrespectable poor whose profligate ways define bad mothering and locate it within the domain of social exclusion or underclass status. Women in the study commonly did not comment on social class directly, however, responses to Jordan and Vicky Pollard provided glimpses into class-inflected perspectives and practices. A 42-year-old respondent living in a rural area comments that there are many young women in the county town that 'look just like' Vicky Pollard, pushing prams, smoking and shouting at their kids, indicating that while the media character may be a caricature of comic excess, the reality exists and is not so far removed from the media portrayal. Many younger respondents, however, found Vicky Pollard 'funny' but unrelated to reality, being quite unlike them or anyone they knew. Such contrasting views suggest that the fault lines of gender and class can be fluid and shifting depending upon who is looking and from what vantage point.

'Bosom Buddies' provided the focus for the generation of other strong emotions. A *Guardian Weekend* feature on women who breastfed their children until they were four or older, with the picture of a breastfeeding child, out of nappies and clearly out of infancy, challenged mothers-to-be in many ways. Many found it difficult to articulate why they found the image disturbing, referring to the phenomena as strange or weird: 'Why would anyone want to carry on for that long?' A more sustained response came from 48-year-old Marion:

> I find that a bit strange. And I wonder whose needs are being met in those scenarios. Because I think socially it's quite difficult for the – if the child thinks that's the norm, and it's very much not the norm, um what are you actually teaching in that process? And I think um – I don't know how they – if there is a father in that scenario how they would feel... in terms of the nutritional value, protection, antibodies all that side of things, I mean even if someone can only breastfeed for a couple of weeks they've still done a lot for that baby in helping with its immune system... Why is that [pointing to image] appropriate for that child? If it's about bonding why is that they way that they are actually bonding?... It doesn't seem quite right to me. It's teaching standards that are not helpful to the child... She [the mother] has not moved on, how can she have a relationship with the child in an appropriate way, an age-appropriate way?

Marion makes her disapproval known on many levels; nutritionally, emotionally and pedagogically it is, for her, the wrong thing to do. The transgressions of 'militant lactators', as they are referred to later in the feature, prompt Marion into an articulation of good mothering as orientated around the needs of the developing child rather than what she sees as the indulgence of a misguided mother. While breastfeeding is generally acknowledged to be the 'best' form of nutrition for the infant, beyond infancy the practice comes to be regarded as temporally and spatially inappropriate – a reviled display of 'matter out of place' (Douglas 1966).

Pregnancy magazines

There is an intense focus on all aspects of the pregnant body throughout pregnancy magazines reflecting, to some extent, the body-beautiful visibility of women within magazines more generally. Pregnancy is no longer regarded as a period of 'confinement', a term that in itself suggests restriction, constraint and time spent away from the public sphere. Rather, pregnancy is to be publicly celebrated and enjoyed. Regularly used phrases and strap lines such as 'bump-tastic', 'blooming marvellous' and 'it's the time of your life' suggest to women that the pregnant body should be displayed, while the burgeoning fashion industry for pregnant women profiled over several pages at the back of each magazine indicates that pregnancy can become a nine-month cat walk in which style and high fashion remain uncompromised by weight gain and the loss of waist line. Furthermore, pregnancy is regarded as an additional reason to look good, pay attention to appearance, to continue to inhabit the feisty, successful, eye-catching and head-turning persona of pre-pregnancy:

> Sex in the City
>
> OK, so you're having a baby (admittedly your greatest achievement to date), but that doesn't mean your smart sassy work wardrobe has to suffer. Show them what you're made of with these killer outfits that will have the office gossips gawping over the coffee machine. (*Pregnancy*, September 2004)

There is the appeal to the fashionable, confident mum-to-be as a unique individual, celebrating her fecundity and enjoying the me-time of pregnancy by pampering herself because she *is* special and this is a special time in her life. A regular feature of *Pregnancy and Birth* entitled 'It's all me, me, me' profiles the latest pamper products for mothers-to-be with the introductory line:

> You're pretty amazing. We reckon that growing a baby is the best excuse ever to spoil yourself or get someone else to do it. (*Pregnancy and Birth*, September 2004)

Magazines call upon pregnant women to indulge themselves as part of the preparation for birth, to write themselves into their to-do list with care-of-the-self activities such as, 'go to the movies, spend time with the girls, get your hair cut, get pampered' (*Prima Baby*, August 2005). Spa breaks and treatments are widely advertised, many of them specifically targeted at mothers-to-be. In an elaboration of this position, many features also suggest that pregnancy is the time for women to strike up a new relationship with their bodies. Women's magazines have a tendency to relate to the body as a project for self-improvement, commonly promoting a range of new regimes in the form of diet and exercise programmes, beauty products and the clever use of clothes and make-up to gain control over an ever-wayward corporeality. Magazines aimed at pregnant women talk back to the regulated body of pre-pregnancy. In a feature calling for women to make ten pregnancy resolutions, loving your body is top of the list:

1. Love your body.
   Hate your big bum, lardy thighs, tiny boobs? Well this is the year you should be celebrating your amazing body and its ability to grow a baby … pregnancy gives us all a break from diet tyranny and while we're not suggesting that you hit the pies, this is the one time in your life that you'll want to see your stomach getting bigger, so enjoy it. (*Pregnancy and Birth*, January 2006)

Loving your body, maintaining pre-pregnancy activities and being kind to yourself become part of a package in which pregnancy is displayed and promoted by the magazines. Loving your body and delighting in getting bigger, however, is short lived. Features on the post-natal body exhort women to 'get your body back in eight weeks', exercise regularly and regain control of weight and shape. The trick to regaining a pre-pregnancy figure is to kick-start the body project as soon as possible after giving birth, focusing once again on regimens of diet and exercise, control and regulation. In these features the ideal of losing the baby weight ('jelly belly' as it's touchingly referred to in one title) and getting back to 'normal' shortly after birth becomes the marker of a successful pregnancy and an accomplished new mother.

First-time pregnancy beckons women into an ever-expanding consumer world of 'maternity' specialist goods and niche marketing, providing products for every stage and every aspect of the maternal experience. Aside from the embodied experience, pregnancy magazines display motherhood though commodities. Commercially produced 'stuff' is everywhere, saturating every magazine in features, advertisements, promotions and consumer guides that take a shameless direct marketing approach. Additionally, most magazines offer free gifts to attract a wider readership.[2] Like other women's magazines, the advertising potential of the title is also a 'value-added' attribute promoted by the publisher. Pregnant body essentials include everyday items such as maternity jeans, nursing bras and moisturising creams, regularly featured as 'must-have' items for expectant mothers. Like other women's magazines, common strategies for profiling products include information on the best and latest 'labour bag luxuries', for example, or the 'beginners guide to toys for newborns', as well as features that put items on trial – 'the best changing bags/pushchairs/baby monitors/stairgates/mobiles' or 'infant carriers at a glance'. Some features take a more sophisticated approach to the 'buy me now' strategy:

Say it with cashmere

Forget flowers. Say congratulations with Daniela Besso's Baby Hamper Service, already a hit with the likes of Claudia Schiffer, Kate Moss and Sadie Frost. Expectant mums deserve a little luxury, and these hampers with their range of cashmere blankets, teddies, cardigans and matching bonnets – all in soft blues, pinks and yellows – are perfect for any special baby occasion. (*Pregnancy*, September 2004)

Here, the appeal relies upon an up-market sensibility and taste signified by the exclusivity of cashmere baby products with celebrity endorsement. Exclusivity, designer labels and personalised products, gift wrapped and delivered to your door, become hallmarks of the special and extraordinary commodities for pregnant women. The 'stylish capsule maternity wardrobe' by Homemummy, for example, offers women a co-ordinating shift dress, trousers and a ballet cardigan, available in black only, in a 'beautifully designed gift box' for £275 (*Junior*, March 2005). The same magazine promoted a designer handbag as 'life changing' in a deft elision between buying a bag and giving birth:

Life changing

A lovely way to celebrate the birth of your new baby is to own this gorgeous Tree of Life embroidered Mother's Bag with the mother-of-pearl button detail £220. It's the latest design by Pink Lining, who make some of the yummiest bags for mummies. Start hinting now ... (*Junior*, March 2005)

In many other features consumption is implicit, associated with lifestyle, desire and taste rather than the direct need to buy. In a special feature on baby showers in *Junior* magazine, Grace tells her story of organising a baby shower for her friend and soon-to-be-mum of twins. Narrated in diary form, Grace documents the arrival of helium balloons, roses, pink champagne, strawberries, cream scones and glamorous guests. For her friend's special send-off Grace has booked her into 'the spa of the moment' for 'some self indulgent "me" time' followed by lunch at Harvey Nicholls, then the baby shower back at her house later in the afternoon. The event is described as 'a big girls" tea party' and a 'rite of passage for new mothers'. The essential ingredients combine organised baby-themed games with gossip, fine food and tasteful gifts:

> Welcome to the celebration of an event that's yet to happen ... The baby shower is the new hot invitation ... 'Demand is very much on the increase,' says Hilary Lewis, director of Babylist, a London-based baby equipment company whose client list includes Gwyneth Paltrow and Elizabeth Hurley ... And this season's hot gifts? Hilary says you can't go wrong with the classic Bill Amberg sling, linen and swiss pique bedding personalised with the baby's name or initials, or a cashmere blanket. (*Junior*, April 2005)

The increased commodification of pregnancy, birth and parenting has extended to areas previously untouched by the commercial sphere. The ante-natal scan, for example, once limited to part of the medical assessment process in early pregnancy has become a commercial venture promoted by several companies as a pre-birth bonding experience for parents-to-be. Widely advertised in the classified ads pages of all the pregnancy magazines, a typical issue will include three to four advertisements from different companies offering three- and four-dimensional non-diagnostic ultrasound scanning at around £100 per session. The companies' promotional materials used in these ads suggest that they are 'scanning to nurture', offering parents-to-be the opportunity to 'capture precious moments' when their baby's may be 'smiling, yawning, blinking, scratching their nose and sucking their fingers' in the womb. The largest company with branches throughout the United Kingdom is Babybond. Providing scans for different stages of pregnancy, Babybond claim to be the creators of the four-dimensional scan 'bonding experience' for women in their 24–32 weeks of pregnancy. Babybond and other ultrasound scanning companies appear to blend romanticism with advanced new technology by suggesting that scans are provided for the purposes of 'bonding, reassurance and foetal wellbeing' (http://www.babybond.com). Like the capsule maternity wardrobe, Babybond products come as a complete package:

> DVD in sleeve, 1 x A4 colour gloss 3D enlargement in photomount, 6 x A6 colour gloss 3D prints, CD-ROM in white, blue or pink Babybond bag, **to take home: £230.** (http://www.babybond.com)

The logic of niche marketing suggests to companies that they pursue an incessant search for ever more specialised and unusual products to appeal to a designated consumer cohort as a necessity for economic survival. The baby market aimed at pregnant women and new parents provides a rich source of opportunity for the creation and marketing of new products. The widely promoted idea that pregnancy is a special time to indulge and be pampered is supplemented by the romantic notion that children are a gift from God. From this perspective, children have a spiritual status placing them close to God and Nature, as the embodiment of innocence, virtue and hope. The legacy of the Romantic movement appears to haunt the present period, particularly in the promotion and marketing of new products.

Tiny toes

You'll be amazed at how quickly your baby's tiny tootsies will grow, but with an extra special momento from Wrightson and Platt you can keep them mini forever!

Using unique techniques, the UK's leading lifecast sculptors will create a perfect cast of your little one's feet in bronze, silver, gold or even glass. The casts are incredibly detailed and will certainly be a talking point with visitors. To make things easier you don't even have to travel as the artists will come to your home. Prices start at £360. (*Pregnancy*, September 2004)

The explicit sentimentality of this artefact, suggesting to parents that they can keep their baby's feet 'mini forever', points to infancy as a desirable and endearing state to be preserved. Whereas photographs, digital film and baby books become tools to document the child's journey from birth through key events in childhood, the lifecast sculpture appears to capture infancy in stasis. Unlike the baby, the bronze feet won't wear shoes, walk, kick or run away, making them simultaneously a preserved memento of babyhood and an object of immobilisation and truncated growth. The preservation of childhood, in this case, falls to parents whose desire to capture the symbolic innocence of their baby's physicality is working in tandem with creative and highly personalised commercial forces.

A further area for the marketing of products focuses upon the home as a transformative site of consumption, as domestic space is rearranged to accommodate the new baby. In this respect magazines tend to profile the creation of a nursery as the room in the house that marks the shift from couple to family. Decorating the nursery is treated as a venture into the future, a space that can be filled with the desires and imaginative projections of becoming new parents. Features on creating a nursery are high on aesthetic appeal, usually filled with an abundance of photographs and little textual commentary. Like other magazines on interior design and home make-overs, features on the nursery commonly conclude with a 'get the look' guide to products and suppliers. Recurrent fashionable themes for nursery décor include white furniture, natural fabrics, pastel and neutral shades and a less-is-more approach to the display of toys, artefacts and childhood memorabilia. Clutter is out – making it a difficult look to maintain for anyone who has young children and limited space. Decorating the nursery highlights parental sensibilities and aspirations; the room itself can become an idealised expression of their tastes and values told through the lens of the environment they choose for their children. The following feature on decorating a boy's nursery points to the significance of style and taste and the ways in which parents draw upon a form of aesthetic capital to respond to the gender of their child and the circumstances of his birth:

A sea and sky theme, illuminated by fairy lights, creates the perfect boy's nursery

After indulging in everything pink and floral for their daughter Isabella-Rose, Grace and Michael Saunders decided to opt for classic French antiques for their second child, Gabriel Sky, adding a nautical theme... Gabriel was born at the peak of a summer heatwave so the aim was to create a room that exudes calm and cool... It retains a masculine feel, with a boat-shaped bookshelf, roughly-hewn boat ornaments and collection of *Tim at Sea* classic stories...

Classic antique pieces are another important element. Key features include a vast French armoire found at a Paris flea market and a charming turn-of-the-century rocking horse, which Grace and Michael spotted – and bartered for – on Portobello Road. And the finishing touch? A watercolour of flowers painted by Gabriel's grandmother. (*Junior*, April 2005)

In this example, decorating a child's bedroom extends beyond the intimacy of the family to become an exercise in class cultural distinction that, like other forms of consumption, speak to wider social formations that point to the link between notions of taste, social class and cultural capital (Bourdieu 1984). Interestingly, the tasteful cosmopolitan couple introduces an intergenerational element into their son's nursery as a 'finishing touch' – a reminder of their creative lineage that is present but not integral to the overall design.

The recurrent themes of the magazines had most appeal for the middle group of women in our study, aged between 25 and 35. Most of these women had timed the birth of their first child to fit around an established career that was possible to 'break' without significant loss of status, the 'right' moment in their personal relationship and the necessary capital resources. Often living a version of the 'pure relationship' (Giddens 1992), the tone, texture and themes of pregnancy magazines appealed to them as resourceful women who had embarked upon pregnancy as a beautiful big adventure that could be personalised to suit their unique style and taste. These women engaged with the birth plan, fashion advice and full immersion in consumer culture; enjoying pregnancy as a project of self-expansion and new consumer experiences. First-time mothers in our older age group, aged 40 to 48 years, were not so ready to be wowed by the magazines. Commonly taking a discerning view of consumption and pregnancy magazines as full of hype and froth, these mature women expressed a desire to retain a strong sense of themselves, untainted by commercial pressure and popular culture.

Preparing for the birth

Towards the end of the interview with first-time mothers-to-be, we asked how they had prepared for the birth of their babies and negotiated making a visual document of their preparations by taking digital photographs. Many women displayed the items they had bought in aesthetic ways, often taking us to a room in the house they have designated as the baby's room. The display of motherhood, however, may start before the preparation of hospital bags or nursery space. In many ways the ultrasonic scan becomes the first visible display of motherhood that commonly exists as a symbolic marker of change, new life and impending motherhood. A professional woman in our study was so pleased about her pregnancy that she pinned the grainy image onto her office door. Other women displayed the images generated at ante-natal appointments in the home, in the kitchen or living room. Another of our respondents arranged all her ultrasonic scan images in a line along the mantel piece like birthday cards, making them the celebratory focal point of the room. While the commercial companies indicate that the scan provides an opportunity for the private experience of nurture and parent-child bonding, the display of these images for women in our study take on the role of 'announcement' and public celebration – speaking to the world rather than the baby. The display of ultrasound scans provides some indication of the intended audience for these images. As a device for making the pregnancy public, displaying the scan facilitates communication with colleagues, family, house guests and even between the couple themselves.

The ways in which women 'wear' their pregnancy provide a further site for the display of the maternal. The embodied display of impending motherhood is shaped in many ways by the personal circumstances in which women find themselves. Women working in competitive and professional masculine environments expressed a wish or a need to conceal their pregnancy, feeling that it compromised their professionalism in the workplace and risked 'letting the side down'. Other women lament the loss of their old selves as their body changes shape and colleagues relate to them in different ways. Hannah, a 26-year-old administrator working in a large car sales company described working in a male environment as affirming a sense of herself as a sexy young thing. Prior to pregnancy she enjoyed attention from men in the workplace, embracing their flattering comments and her ability to exercise her femininity to get what she wanted. Being pregnant has changed all that. As workplace relations reconfigure, she has been upset by 'fatty' jokes, hasn't taken to maternity wear as it disrupts her image of herself and can't wait to get her figure back. For younger women becoming pregnant in their teens, the body remains a source of pride and shame. Displaying the tummy can be an act of defiance, a 'What you gonna do about it?' flash of resistance designed to shock adults around them. For other young women, aware of the negative ways in which they may be perceived, the bump may be something they privately enjoy but seek to conceal in public spaces.

For all our respondents, preparing for the birth could be both a simple, practical matter of being ready and an elaborate baby audit of imagining, doing and projecting. In all cases the 'situation' of motherhood comes into sharp focus as personal circumstances and family resources shape the contours of the pregnancy and birth experience in consequential ways. The grandmother of a teenage mother expressed concern with the way her 15-year-old granddaughter was preparing for the birth of her baby:

> I went in to Kim's bedroom one day and...she had this big suitcase, from under her bed, and I says to her: 'What are you doing?' And it was full of baby things, 'Oh I'm taking notes on what I've got', and I says, 'Why, is that so you don't duplicate anything?' 'Oh no I just like doing this.'...I just thought it was funny, why would she want to take a note of what was in the suitcase?...I mean she knew what was in there and I always, my interpretation of it was that it was like a child with a doll, and I think that's what she thought it was going to be, and all of a sudden this baby comes along and, my god, what a responsibility.

Another teenage mother found herself preparing for the birth of her baby in a local authority residential care facility for young mothers. Interviewing her in this setting a few weeks before the birth prompted [in the researcher] a mixture of feelings and an acute awareness of her limited resources:

> Sophie meets me and takes me to her unit. It is very small – a kitchen/lounge and one bedroom with just enough room for a single bed, a chest of drawers and nothing else... I felt that it was compact and had everything she needed but that it was also an infantilising space for a young mother-to-be. The bedroom in particular seemed to emphasise her youthful status as a child who was expecting a child. It was a girl's room, there was a cartoon motif on her duvet – it's not *My Little Pony* but it reminds me of that. A Moses basket on a stand and a baby relaxer lined the corridor-like space next to the bed... she had bought a few basics – nappies, sterilising kit, vests and socks. (Fieldnotes, 22.8.05)

We found that women in the 25- to 35-years age group were more likely to embrace the opportunity to display motherhood. Having more than a suitcase or a single bedroom to work with, pregnancy for these women gave them license to develop an expanded version of self that commonly incorporated the reorganisation of domestic space. Pregnancy signalled an opportunity to get everything around the house 'sorted', giving the couple a joint project anchored in the family rather than work. Women spoke of having the kitchen done, putting in radiators and redecorating as well as preparing the baby's room. Naomi, a 35-year-old professional summed up the approach by telling us that, before the pregnancy, they had put up with things being half done and other things not working. Having a baby has motivated her and her partner to be 'housey', prioritising their personal lives by making sure that the domestic space is prepared for the arrival of the baby. Informed by pregnancy magazines, baby books and websites, many women chose products with care and reported putting time and energy into finding the 'right' baby buggy, baby gym or nursery furniture. Taking pleasure in the exercise of consumption in new markets, first-time pregnancy is presented as a time when it is *necessary* for couples to re-evaluate, change and spend.

The creation of a nursery offers the possibility for an elaborate display of motherhood as parents-to-be create a special place within the home for the new baby. Women in our study presented this space in various states of 'readiness' from bare walls splurged with paint pot colours and decorating mess to pristine and beautifully finished rooms. The new baby's room usually spoke, consciously and unconsciously, to the desires of the maternal as women sought to surround the child with the things that appeared important to them as a new family. While some women took the view that the child is entering our world as a couple, others worked to create a unique environment for their baby. Choosing primary colours or pastels, gender-specific items or neutral pieces, purpose-made nursery furniture or customised pieces all pointed to the significance of the maternal project as an investment in shaping the world of the baby in ways that are imbued with emotional connections. Hannah, a 26-year-old woman, spoke of decorating the nursery as a way of displaying the things that were important to her and, she hoped, would become important to her child. Hannah wanted to keep the memory of her dead mother alive and wanted her child to know her by creating a presence out of absence. She placed a framed photograph of her mother in the nursery and planned to talk about her routinely, to share the activities her mother enjoyed and to take her child to visit the grave regularly. On the radiator in magnetic letters it says, 'Mummy and Daddy love you'. Working to create family bonds and maintain intergenerational connections became key features in the way Hannah prepared for the birth of her child.

Conclusion

In this chapter we have presented an account of the three ways in which motherhood was displayed during the course of a research project on the transition to first-time motherhood. Discussing the concept of motherhood as display across the study, the chapter explored the visual prompt material used in interview, pregnancy magazines and, finally, the ways in which women prepared for the birth of their first child. Viewed collectively, the idea that motherhood can be displayed has points of resonance and points of departure with Finch's (2007) notion of displaying families. Motherhood as an identity seeks recognition within the couple relationship and the wider family. The 'social reality' of becoming a mother engages women in a range of practices that involve expressive forms of display which seek social recognition. Examples discussed in the chapter point to the constitution of an audience for acts of recognition and the different fractions with which first-time mothers-to-be may be in dialogue as they embark upon a maternal project that creates 'family'. Pregnancy itself is imbued with meaning that is class coded and culturally specific. What pregnant women wear, buy and do become the prism for intensified forms of display that cross the boundaries of public and private. These practices are inevitably connected to wider landscapes of class, representation and consumption, drawn upon by pregnant women to define a sense of themselves as new mothers-to-be.

Defining an emergent identity simultaneously involves differentiation from others who occupy the same status but may not share the same approach to it. Celebrity pregnancies, comedic characters and breastfeeding practices demonstrated some of the ways in which pregnant women distinguished themselves from each other in the process of shaping a maternal identity for themselves. Our approach suggests the importance of understanding displays of family in relation to the wider circuits of cultural meaning that both incite and constrain these performances. We also depart from Finch's focus on display as an attempt to consolidate family practices over time and space, suggesting the importance of understanding the consumption practices of first-time mothers as acts of imagination. In the reconfiguration of domestic space to accommodate the new baby, women and couples engage in the creation of an idealised environment that brings into being the fantasies, desires and imaginative projections of a *family-in-the-making*.

Notes

1. The Making of Modern Motherhood: Memories, Identities, Representations research project (RES 148–25-0057) was funded by the Economic and Social Research Council between 2005 and 2008 as part of the Identities and Social Action research programme, (www.identities.ac.uk). The project was directed by Rachel Thomson and Mary Jane Kehily and involved Lucy Hadfield and Sue Sharpe. A subsequent stage of the study, The Dynamics of Motherhood, has been funded by the ESRC as part of the Timescapes initiative (www.timescapes.leeds.ac.uk).
2. Splash mats, baby cutlery, name books, t-shirts, story book CDs, baby blankets, teat and soother sets and baby bath puppets are just some of the freebies collected over the study period.

5

'It's Just Not Good for a Man to be Interested in Other People's Children': Fathers, Public Displays of Care and 'Relevant Others'

Andrea Doucet

Introduction

Sean (1992; Cambridge, England; stay-at-home father of two):

I was passing a postman cycling by and I was pushing the push chair and holding Luke's hand and I thought he's given me a sort of 'What a big sissy. A big sissy'! You know that may have been my response because you do interpret things according to your own level of comfort or discomfort to a certain extent. And then on an another occasion, I walked past some builders just round the corner and one of them was knocking a wall down and turned to his friend and he said: `That's what you ought to do'.

Archie (2002; Ottawa, Canada; stay-at-home father of two):

Initially, when Brad was in kindergarten, this woman comes up and introduces herself and says 'I am a little embarrassed but I am coming to check you out'. I said 'Okay'. She said 'My daughter came home and told me about this man hanging around the schoolyard reading stories to the kids'. She said 'I hope you are not offended'. At this point I am used to it. I said 'Isn't it interesting, if a kid came home and said a mom is reading to kids in the yard, you would say "Isn't that nice", and wouldn't give it another thought'. She admitted that was true.

Christopher (2009; Boston, United States; stay-at-home father of four):

You know like when I first found out that I was going to be staying at home my friends all made their little comments... I don't care but they definitely all made their smart Alec comments that oh you know – 'Mr. Mom' or whatever. Yeah so um so that is everybody's initial reaction but it is changing times. It's amazing if I tried to do this or we did this fifteen years ago I would look like a freak show probably. You know a dad walking around with four little kids. I'm already a freak show as it is.

This chapter is rooted in two decades of research on mothering and fathering and gender and care work in households where women are the shared or primary breadwinners and where fathers are the shared or primary caregivers. My research, conducted mainly in Canada (2000 to 2009), as well as in the United Kingdom (1992 to 1995) and in the United States (2008 to 2010), has included a series of interlocking qualitative research projects where I have personally interviewed over 250 women and men, including a small case study of men and women who have been followed over the course of a decade in Canada (Doucet 2006a, forthcoming). Across three distinct countries, I have spoken to men, as well as women, about the personal and political challenges and opportunities that recur when 'doing family' means reversing or re-adjusting what are still dominant and hegemonic conceptions of male breadwinners and female caregivers.

My sustained interest in this research area began two decades ago when one father's story stayed with me as a compelling narrative of the difficulties for women and men who were charting different ways of 'doing gender' and 'doing family'. The first quote at the beginning of this chapter from British stay-at-home dad Sean, articulated twenty years ago on how he felt that he was viewed as a 'big sissy' by a postman and a male construction worker, pulled me into the puzzle of what enables and constrains men's involvement in care work. Moreover, it was Sean's narrative, and many more since then, that instigated my thinking on how community responsibilities, enacted in spaces that combine households and communities, are an integral part of the 'doing' of family and the social judgements of families.

Janet Finch's new concept of 'display' provides a further way of conceptualising the challenges faced by mothers and fathers who attempt to 'do' gender and family differently. As indicated in the quotes that open this chapter, men who care for children repeatedly mention how their 'displays' of care work, as well as of alternative family forms and non-hegemonic masculinities, are scrutinised and surveilled by others; specifically, men can often find themselves under a community spotlight, where they feel treated as 'sissies', potential pedophiles, or a 'freak show'.

Three of Finch's (2007) key contentions about the display of family are employed in this chapter. First, I draw from her point that narratives and objects are tools for displaying family. Second, build on her argument about how displays of family involve 'the conveying of meaning through social interaction and the acknowledgment of this by relevant others' (Finch 2007: 77). There is, moreover, an on-going 'process of seeking legitimacy (which) necessarily entails displaying one's chosen family relationships to relevant others and having them accepted' (Finch 2007: 71). My third argument extends my second point about public legitimacy as I further develop Finch's point (2007: 72) about how it is important 'to think about *degrees of intensity* in the need for display, depending on circumstances'.

Methodological, theoretical and empirical locations

While this chapter is rooted broadly in two decades of research on mothering and fathering, it is specifically rooted in four qualitative research studies carried out over the past ten years (2000 to 2010) in Canada, as well as more recently in the United States. The first study (2000 to 2005) of fathers who are primary caregivers (single fathers and/or stay-at home fathers) included in-depth interviews with over one hundred fathers and with fourteen heterosexual couples (see Doucet 2006a). The second (2004 to 2008) is a qualitative research study with twenty-six Canadian couples (twenty-five heterosexual and one gay) where the father has taken some parental leave (see McKay and Doucet 2010), while the third research project (2004 to 2009) focused on transitions to new fatherhood for a diverse sample of fathers, mainly gay fathers and immigrant fathers, from across Canada; focus groups were conducted with fifty fathers and in-depth interviews with twenty fathers (Doucet 2009a). Finally, this chapter is influenced by my current research and writing on Canadian and American households (2008 to 2010) where women are primary breadwinners and men are primary or shared caregivers (Doucet, forthcoming). Across all of these studies is a small case study of men and women who have been followed over the course of a decade in

Canada (Doucet 2006a, forthcoming). While the majority of individuals interviewed are lower middle class and middle class, of varied white ethnicities, heterosexual, and living with dependent children, my projects also include diversity across class, race and sexuality, across Canada and more recently in the United States.

The empirical context that informs my work is one where there has been some evidence of fathers' increasing participation in the care of children in many Western countries. In the case of Canada, its social terrain is characterised by the rising labour-force participation of mothers of young children and gradual increases in the numbers of stay-at-home fathers; the latter have increased 25 per cent over the past decade so that, on average, men constitute one-tenth of stay-at-home parents (Statistics Canada 2002). The proportion of lone-parents who are male has also increased over the past three decades; between 1976 and 2008, the proportion of male single parents increased from 14 per cent of all lone-parents to 20 per cent (Statistics Canada LFS, unpublished data 2009). It is also worth noting that women are primary breadwinners in nearly one-third of Canadian two-earner families (Sussman and Bonnell 2006).[1] Over the past ten years, fathers' participation in infant care has also increased, partly as a result of policy changes in parental-leave provisions.[2]

Theoretically, my work has long-standing roots in socialist feminist work on the importance of valuing unpaid work (Luxton 1980/2010; Luxton and Vosko 1998); a focus on gender relations, men and masculinities (Connell 2005); and feminist theoretical and philosophical writing on the connections between care work and social justice (Held 1993, 2005; Okin 1989; Ruddick 1995; Young 1990, 1997). For over a decade, I have argued for a conceptualisation of care that is intrinsically relational, embodied, embedded in daily practice, linked with what symbolic interactionists would call 'moral identities' (Finch 2007; Finch and Mason 1993), framed by varied kinds of time (biographical, generational and historical), and articulated in domestic and community spaces (see Doucet 2000, 2001, 2006a, 2006b, 2009a, 2009b). I agree with many feminist and family scholars who have argued that gender *should not matter* to the ways in which care is undertaken and, indeed, that men can and do take on care work in ways that can be viewed as indistinguishable from that enacted by their female partners (see Biblarz and Stacey 2010; Doucet 2006a; Ranson 2010; Smith, J. 2009). Nevertheless, while men can and do partake in childcare, I have also argued that there has been little shift in the *responsibility* for care work. As argued in this chapter, at least part of the puzzle for this continuing resistance in gendered divisions of domestic responsibility and care work lies in the differing pressures exerted on men and women who display their care of children in community settings.

Displaying families through narratives and through family objects

I am in agreement with Finch that 'narratives are one tool which can be used in displaying families' (2007: 78). She also maintains that 'a fundamental driving force in presenting families to an external audience is to convey the message "this is my family and it works"' (Finch 2007: 70; see also Finch and Mason 1993). In addition to how families can be displayed through narratives, there are, as Finch argues (2007: 77), 'ways in which such displays are supported' by particular domestic objects or what 'we might think of as "tools" for display'. Several examples emerge from my research on how fathers display particular conceptions of family through narratives as well as through domestic objects. Four examples will be discussed in this section.

Display of family and fathering through heroic narratives

First, in relation to display through narratives, my research on fathers as primary caregivers reveals that 'heroic narratives' are often employed by men in order to display their families as ones that work, in part because of their extraordinary efforts towards making them work in social environments that often assume men's incompetence in caregiving. Heroic narratives are defined as ones that are framed partly by a telling of a 'heroic tale' that is 'oriented around some heroic struggle' (Presser 2004: 92; see also Doucet 2008). Two examples of such heroic displays of family are mentioned here.

The first is from Dennis, an ethnic minority and low-income single father of a 10-year-old girl. In his interview with me in 2003, he told a story of a father facing considerable strain and difficulty as he balanced a heavy debt load, long hours working as a cook in a fast-food restaurant, a highly conflictive relationship with the mother of his daughter who lived two thousand miles away, and living in a small apartment that he and his daughter shared with two male boarders. Sitting with me in his kitchen with a basket of perfectly folded laundry beside him, two constant themes in his interview were how he said he wanted to be on the Oprah Winfrey show and how people kept telling him: 'I can't believe your daughter is so good. I've never seen a kid this good'. However, such exuberant statements of believed, or hopeful, heroism were out of sync with much of his narrative as well as with my sense of this father, as gleaned from the interview setting, and from the detailed field notes that my research assistant and I took after the interview.

Looking back to this interview, and drawing on Finch, I would argue that Dennis wanted to participate in my study because he wanted to display that his version of family worked. Moreover, his desire to appear on Oprah and his constant references to others' comments on how his daughter was 'so good' could be viewed as instances of displaying and legitimating family through narrative. My case study of Dennis also revealed objects of family display; I refer here to the basket of perfectly folded laundry which he had beside his chair. Dennis deliberately displayed this as part of his family life while other less noticeable aspects of his home and family life – such as the peeling wallpaper in the kitchen or the entrance of the two male boarders who lived in his basement – were objects and subjects that Dennis tried to downplay and, indeed, not to display.

A second example of a 'heroic narrative' can be illustrated through the case of Mick, a 45-year-old transport truck driver and the sole-custody father of a 16-year-old daughter. Mick was jolted into becoming a primary caregiving father when Mary Kate's mother left when her daughter was three years old. Interviewed in 2003, he told the story of how he learned of this state of affairs when he was out of town and received a distressed phone call from his father who lived with Mick's family. As he described it, Mick then drove his transport truck over five hundred miles back to his home to find his pre-kindergarten daughter standing on the street wearing 'her little summer dress with the flowers'. In his words:

> Mary Kate came home from school. She was in pre-kindergarten and her mother was not home. She was supposed to be there. My father called me. So I went to Windsor, I dropped the truck's trailer, and I came from Windsor with no trailer, just my own

truck. I came as fast as I could. When I came down the street she was in her little summer dress with the flowers. And she was standing there holding onto the street sign on our lawn. And my Dad was on the verandah, sitting there watching. I promised Mary Kate that never would I let this happen again. I parked my truck and ended up selling my truck. I never went back on the road again. I promised her that I would do that. That's when it started.

Mick's narrative was filled with heroic statements about how he 'had to do it' and how he was 'going to stick with my commitment, my damn commitment':

There is no way that I would have said – 'Go to Children's Aid or something like that.' Her mother is not going to do it. Well damn, I am going to do it. I'm not going to let someone else do it. It is my job. It was a choice that I had to make. I knew that I had to do it. It was never a question. I was there and I had to do it. There were days when I used to sit there and cry when Mary Kate was sleeping and wonder. It wasn't a case of – 'Am I doing it right or wrong'? It was – 'I had to do it. I am going to get through it.' [...] It is my responsibility. I took a commitment and I am going to stick with my commitment, my damn commitment'.

He also constantly referred to the misfit between 'my transport truck in the yard' and 'folding Mary Kate's underwear'; this counter-posing of a strong masculine and an equally strong feminine image was meant to convey a deliberate display of how, against many odds, he was still capable of such heroic efforts. Mick and Dennis, both low-income and sole-custody fathers, used the interview process, and the heroic narratives produced therein, to convey the idea that their family forms 'worked'.

Display of gendered domestic space

A second example of the display of family through narrative and domestic objects emerges from my observations across two decades of visiting couples in their homes. Women are more likely to display family and domestic life, as well as 'good mothering' through the presentation of a clean and ordered home, while men are more likely to display their place in the family and their role as a good father through their work in household renovation. That is, domestic space and domestically acquired identities have different connotations for women and men (see also Young 1997).

One example of this is provided by Kyle, a Canadian stay-at-home father interviewed in 2004, who made a point to let me know that his wife Carol 'did the vacuuming before she left for work today because she knew you were coming to interview me'. While Kyle admitted that he was 'fanatical' about cleaning as well as a 'neat freak', he did not worry about the presentation of their home to others to the extent that his wife did. He confessed that he liked to keep the kitchen clean because he was the one who did most of the cooking: 'If I'm going to cook, I have to do the shopping. If I'm going to cook, I have to make sure the counters are clean. I suffered many years ago from two bouts of salmonella; I don't intend to do that again'. In contrast, his wife Carol was more concerned about the house being clean, especially when *it is seen by others*. He gave the example of people coming to assess the house:

> I was in the home show, met up with one of the real estate agents who offered to do an assessment. I said – 'Oh, ya, sure come on over at such and such a time'. Carol was absolutely in a tizzy over that because, could she guarantee that the house would be perfectly clean when someone comes in to deliberately look in every corner? And I said – '*So what?*'.

Across the four studies that inform this chapter, many stay-at-home fathers reconstruct the meanings of work and home to include unpaid self-provisioning work (Pahl 1984; Wallace and Pahl 1985), specifically 'male self-provisioning activities' which include 'building, renovation... carpentry, electrical repairs and plumbing, furniture making, decorating, constructing doors and window frames, agricultural cultivation for own use, repairing vehicles' (Mingione 1988: 560–1). While some of these can be viewed as masculine hobbies, which these men would have likely picked up from their fathers or male peers, these are also activities which display or justify men's masculinity and which seem to alleviate some of the discomfort men feel with giving up breadwinning.

Displaying 'happy families' in interviews

Building again on Finch's point that 'a fundamental driving force in presenting families to an external audience is to convey the message "this is my family and it works"' (Finch 2007: 73; see also Finch and Mason 1993), I would argue that men and women often engage in such displays of 'happy families' in interview settings. That is, in couple interviews, there is a tendency, as Duncombe and Marsden (1993) astutely pointed out many years ago, to present the 'we are ever so happy really' face to the interviewer and, more generally, to their social worlds.

Recognising this persistent tendency in family research, while also echoing John Law's broader point (2004) that particular methods produce particular social realities, I maintain that the close connections between issues of deeply held 'moral' identity and how families are displayed and judged by others require that sustained attention is paid to the methods we use in family research. One commonly used strategy is that of interviewing different family members who can provide different windows into family realities (see Edwards et al. 2006; Mauthner and Doucet 2003). Even where couples are the centre of the analysis, interviewing both couples and individuals can provide different angles on family life while longitudinal interviewing over time can pull forth and reconfigure varied understandings from participants (see McLeod and Thomson 2009). Finally, an approach that focuses on networks of relations (see Hansen 2005) can provide wider understandings of the meanings of family life that disrupt the smooth displays provided by some participants. In this vein, Karen Hansen's path-breaking book *Not So Nuclear Families: Class, Gender and Networks of Care* (2005) moves away from traditional interview studies of 'independent individuals' to focus on 'connected individuals who are part of a parent's network of care' (2005: 13). Working from four in-depth case studies, Hansen 'focuses on a network, a web of people, rather than on a collection of separate individuals' as she probes 'the interaction and interpretations and meaning people assign to their involvements and interactions with other people' (2005: 13).

Finch also maintains that display is different from performance in that the audience is not passive and indeed participates in the ongoing construction of meaning. She writes (2007: 77): 'the concepts of performance/performativity – and the associated concepts of actors and audiences – are not adequate in themselves for understanding how "family" meanings are conveyed'. While I agree with the general tenor of this argument, I would, however, argue that methodologically there can be a performative element that recurs in interviews so that interviews can be used as vehicles to display particular understandings of self and family life to interviewers and to the re-telling of those stories to others (see Doucet 2008; Presser, 2004).

Displaying masculinities

In addition to displaying family in their narratives, men also work to display their masculinity in appropriate ways that resonate with hegemonic conceptions of masculinities. What seems very clear in most fathers' narratives is their determination to distinguish themselves *as men*, as heterosexual males, and as fathers, *not* as mothers (Doucet 2006a). Throughout my two decades of interviewing fathers, I have heard recurring interjections by fathers that confirm how they are adamant to 'display' hegemonic masculinity in which the devaluation of the feminine is a central part (see Connell 2005). For example, in a focus group with stay-at-home fathers held in 2000, Sam, a stay-at-home father of two for five years, interjected several times, half jokingly: 'Well we're still *men*, aren't we?' Several years later, another stay-at-home father, Mitchell, made several pointed references to how he often worked out at a gym and enjoyed 'seeing the women in Lycra'. These men's words support what theorists of work have underlined about men working in non-traditional or female-dominated occupations (such as nursing or elementary school teaching) and how they must actively work to dispel the idea that they might be gay, un-masculine, or not men (Fisher and Connell 2002; Sargent 2000; Williams 1992).

From my research on fathers who are actively involved in care work, I have argued that these men are thus attempting to carve out their own paternal and masculine identities within spaces traditionally considered maternal and feminine (Doucet 2005). A recent example of this tendency comes from an interview in 2009 with Sally, an engineer who is the primary breadwinner in her family; she notes that one difference between her experiences at home with two pre-school children and that of her husband Wilson was the following:

> Wilson was more about doing work and bringing Ryan along. So he would take him to like a job site where he was fixing someone's

radiator and he'd either bring a couple of toys or a book or let Ryan have a toy wrench. So Ryan went with him for the first couple of years to jobs. Or he was renovating the basement at the time so they would just renovate the basement together. The cutest videos of Ryan are where he is in diapers with a power drill – drilling holes in a piece of plywood that Wilson had set up for him.

Public displays that are 'legitimate' and managing displays

Finch (2007: 71) points out that 'the process of seeking legitimacy necessarily entails displaying one's chosen family relationships to relevant others and having them accepted'. While she relies mainly on examples of non-heterosexual families, it is also the case that in heterosexual two-parent families as well as in single parent families, particular displays of family life are rendered more palatable than others. That is, families who adopt differing patterns around care and breadwinning can also face scrutiny. From my research, there are three recurring examples of how fathers seek public legitimacy as they work to display the acceptability of themselves as carers while simultaneously attempting to refrain from disruptive displays in community settings of their unconventional families. Specifically, my research demonstrates that fathers without female partners often work particularly diligently to convey that they are suitable caregivers and that they are 'doing family' in socially acceptable ways. Furthermore, I argue that some fathers need to *manage* their displays and that this is especially marked for fathers who display alternative masculinities, notably low-income or unemployed fathers, gay fathers, and fathers caring for the children of others.[3]

Low-income or unemployed fathers

To be placed in a position of primary caregiver without having achieved success as a breadwinner signals something out of sync with what many communities consider as a socially acceptable 'moral' identity for a male and for a father.[4] My argument here is that fathers need to work to display both their masculinity as well as their family in socially acceptable ways. From my study on fathers as primary caregivers and my recent work on women who are primary breadwinners, I would argue that fathers without jobs or those in low-income jobs, especially single fathers, can be viewed with particular suspicion within communities. For example, Henry, who was periodically out of work, highlighted how his lower social class and frequent unemployed status was one of the reasons why his house was not viewed as an acceptable option for his daughter's sleepovers:

> My daughter sleeps over at a friend's place right across the street, and her friend never comes back. I push it in the sense that it isn't fair. I actually try to mention it to the parents and stuff, but it's no big deal. They live in a nice big detached house. The girl mentioned has two full sets of parents that both live in nice big detached houses with multiple cars, or that kind of thing. And I live in this townhouse co-op place.

In contrast, Jacob, a physician-in-training, noted that sleepovers were never a problem at his house, either for his two sons or for his 11-year-old daughter. He reflected on how this and his acceptance as a frequent helper in his children's schools may be rendered unproblematic, partly because his occupation is one of high status:

> I am involved in the school. I help out on field trips. I go in and help to read whatever I can. I am also the head-lice coordinator. Once or twice a month I go and look at heads! I know the teachers and the principal and a lot of the kids. I also know them from ringette and hockey. I feel very accepted. [...] Being a doctor may be part of it. It might be different if I was a plumber.

Stay-at-home fathers fare slightly better, although not working can still spark community alarm bells if it seems that the father may have lost his job and is not in his caring situation due to a family 'choice'. For example, Theo, who left his job in the high tech sector told me in 2004: 'Everybody assumed I was laid off'. James, a gay and divorced father who took a four-month paternity leave also commented in 2004:

> I think there is still a stigma for men with staying-at-home particularly around other men. I can't tell you how many times people ask as a first liner; 'So, what do you do for a living?' When I answered 'I stay-at-home', most wondered – 'Well what happened?'

What is at issue here is how a key resource of hegemonic masculinity – that of social status acquired through being a family provider, especially in a high income or high status profession – helps to increase fathers' ability to display socially acceptable fathering within both families and communities, while also cushioning them from being viewed with suspicion. What is playing out here are the links between hegemonic masculinity and earning. In effect, the economically unsuccessful male caring for children represents a form of double jeopardy because he is judged as being a *'failed* male' (that is, not a breadwinner) (Thorne 1993: 161) and as a *'deviant* man' (that is, a primary caregiver). On the other hand, a male who is visibly providing economically for his family, or has temporarily left a career that allows him to do this, is involved in more acceptable displays of both masculinity and fathering practice.

Gay fathers and the display of heterosexuality as a 'resource of masculinity'

The constitution of gay families is incredibly diverse with varied configurations of men raising children with other men and/or with other women, often across several households (see Dunne 2001). What emerges from my interviews with a small sample of sixteen gay fathers over the past decade is that space and community setting matter for the public legitimacy of these diverse family forms. Nevertheless, issues of social acceptability are especially acute for gay fathers, many of whom can face extra scrutiny over their role with children. They can confront 'multiple jeopardy' (King 1990, cited in Ward 2004: 82) in that intersections of gender, class, sexuality, as well as geographical location can facilitate particular kinds of exclusion and social judgement for some gay fathers. One good example of this was expressed by Jean Marc, a French-Canadian, 43-year-old gay and divorced father of seven-year-old twin boys whom I interviewed in 2004. He lived in a small town in Ontario and his ex-wife had sole custody. Although he had taken a four-month parental leave when his twins were infants and was very involved in their lives, his 'coming out' led to him being shunned by his wife and her family:

> I thought that she would be accepting and that she would understand this. It was the opposite. The kids were removed from the house. I was told to get out. I cried for a week. I was clinically

depressed for quite some time. What really helped me was Gay Fathers of Toronto. And I got some counseling. It really hurt me that Monique didn't want joint custody ... I think she was absolutely terrified of me taking the kids to Toronto and maybe bringing them into some kind of immoral lifestyle.

Even though Jean Marc gradually became more involved with his children over time, he remained disinclined to 'come out' to the school and the wider community because he feared that if community members, particularly teachers, knew that he was gay, it would lead them to think he was 'riff raff off the street':

I think it's important that I go and meet their teachers. I have not met any of their teachers yet (long sigh). [...] I am perhaps somewhat timid. I don't know. I just didn't know what to expect. It's a situation where their teacher is married to a police officer in the town. Everybody knows me. I will go. [...] I want them to know that- 'Hey I am a good father. I am involved. And you may have heard that I am gay and that is absolutely correct. But I am not some riff raff off the street'.

Several gay fathers were less concerned about managing their displays of fathering and the key factor here was the greater community acceptance of diversity in parenting, combined with organisations that have provided both support and information for gay fathers in their 'coming out' processes. Such resources are more available in larger urban settings where there is a rich heterogeneity of lifestyles, and a positive acknowledgement of such choices. For example, Bernard (interviewed in 2005), who lived in Toronto and shared custody of a four-year-old son with two lesbian mothers, found his situation palatable because 'there are other children at the school who have two dads or two moms. So he is not alone there. We live in a progressive area'. Similar stories of acceptance were told by Ray and Carson (interviewed in 2004 and again in 2006) who adopted two infants over the course of four years and were 'embraced by the community'. What is demonstrated here is that in order to facilitate family and fathering displays that are treated as 'normal' or acceptable, gay fathers often have to demonstrate that they can blend into parenting settings so that gender and sexuality lose such critical significance.

Fathers and the children of others

Across two decades of interviewing fathers who are primary or shared primary caregivers, I have noticed that a dominant father-daughter narrative revolves around the hidden, unspoken sense of unease that fathers can face when they are caring for the children of others. For example, this sense of unease can occur when fathers are babysitting, are caring for children where issues of undressing are involved, and are supervising girls' sleepovers.

Babysitting children is an issue that has come up often in my interviews with men and is a theme that arose in my first study on mothers and fathers in Britain in the early 1990s (Doucet 1995). More recently, in 2003, a Canadian stay-at-home father, Jess, spoke about how he could only babysit the children of a very small group of friends and that this barrier was caused by his gender: 'It's kind of bad for men to be interested in other children'.

Caring for children where it involves physical tasks such as changing diapers or young children's clothes also leads men to manage their displays of care so as to avoid scrutiny of their alternative family arrangements around caregiving. Again, this theme is carried over a long trail of interviews with fathers over many years. A recent example comes from David, a stay-at-home father of three in a suburb outside Toronto, Canada. While he was clearly the primary parent of their three children while his wife Bonnie worked long hours as a pharmacist, he still found that there was one area where he had to manage his displays of care. He says:

> Well right now, like changing Molly [7 years old], bathing her, it just doesn't sit right. Or her friends come over, right. Get undressed, put on costumes and stuff and they call me for help. It doesn't sit right.

Finally, girls' sleepovers are the window through which many men see the need to be very careful around their teen daughters and their friends. As Ryan, a sole-custody father of a son and a 12-year-old girl put it in 2003:

> I have purposefully not had anybody to sleep over, especially girls, because I'm really leery of the possibility that somebody might think something bad.

Intensity in display

My third and final argument on fathers' display of family and care work is informed by Finch's point (2007: 72) about how it is important 'to think about *degrees of intensity* in the need for display, depending on circumstances'. While Finch (2007: 72) points to how these changed circumstances can be when 'new individuals – new relationships – come into the picture', she also notes that they can involve particular changes such as when 'a woman who has previously focused on caring for children takes a full-time job'. Set against hegemonic conceptions around gendered paid and unpaid work, many women and men still point to how they are judged and observed, and thus there is a constant sense of intensity to their displays of family. The 'intensity' is therefore not related to change in particular family circumstances but a disjuncture between what is expected of men and women and an intense need to display that 'this is my family and it works' (Finch 2007: 75).

I argue here that the need to display that family 'works' is especially intense in relation to the gendered arrangements for the care of infants. Quite simply, it is assumed that women will care for infants and will take time off from work, either through unpaid leave or through maternity or parental leave.

Fathers caring for infants

Across the two decades that I have been researching fathering, the issue of men caring for infants recurs as one that invites scrutiny, and well as public judgement. Craig, for example, a Canadian stay-at-home dad with twin sons, one of whom has physical disabilities (interviewed in 2002), reflected on how an on-going issue for him as a father is that 'the incompetence thing comes into play', and how social onlookers 'very much want to make sure that the babies are okay'. He remembers how he was often 'approached with offers of help. It was very much like the incompetent father needing a woman's help to get the job done'.

Peter, a stay-at-home father of two sons (interviewed twice in 2003 and again in 2010) also points to how community sentiments of assumed incompetence on the part of fathers are particularly strong with young or preverbal children because onlookers may worry about the baby's care, while also assuming that the father is a secondary, and less competent, carer; he also highlights how this perception wanes as the children grow older:

> When he was a tiny baby, there was always that sense that I was babysitting rather than taking care of my child like I do every-day – where I had to understand his wants and needs because he can't speak. That's where I felt it was very different from women. There was a bit of an assumption that I felt like I was just tiding things over until the *real mother* showed up, or the *person who really knew what they were doing* would show up.

At the end of his interview in 2003, Peter gave a frank assessment of the social acceptability of fathers as carers:

> Even in a society where people believe that men and women are equal and can do just about everything, they don't really believe that men can do this with a baby, especially a really tiny baby.

Women giving up the care of infants

Assumptions about men as secondary caregivers also filter into men's desires to take parental leave and women's decisions to give up some of their parental-leave time to fathers. That is, when women give up primary caregiving to focus on breadwinning, either by not taking all of their allotted leave quota or by prioritising work over caregiving, they also must work to dispel community judgements that they are not doing family in appropriate ways. For example, when Arianna (interviewed with her husband Brandon in 2006) returned to her job as a schoolteacher, she was confronted by disapproval from her colleagues:

> I think it's becoming more common, but it's not common at all, really... People kind of think... that somehow that I'm not as good a mother cause I wanted to go back to work and I'm ok with letting my husband stay home. It was kind of like, 'Ok, that's weird'... (It was) mostly women.

This systemic sense that infant care is women's care is strongly demonstrated in my co-authored work on couples' decision making around parental leave (see Doucet et al. 2009a; McKay and Doucet 2010). While Canadian policy now has a six-month gender-neutral entitlement that is available to both mothers and fathers, many parents still refer to this as 'maternity leave' and there is a strong sense on the part of both mothers and fathers that this is 'her leave' (McKay and Doucet 2010). When such dominant norms are violated, families feel an intense pressure to display that their family still 'works' even though they have gone against the grain of strongly rooted norms around infant care.

Fathers in child-centered spaces

There is an intensity of display required of fathers who find themselves having to work against community notions that men do not always belong in child-centred community spaces. The quotations from men at the beginning of this chapter, spanning two decades and three national contexts, aptly capture this sense of community judgement and surveillance that men can experience when they take on care work. As indicated in these fathers' narratives, men who take on full-time care work can sometimes find themselves under a community spotlight where they feel that they are viewed as 'sissies', potential pedophiles or 'freak shows'. It is important to note that class, sexuality, locality, as well as time also mediate community judgements around men and care. There is thus some intensity to the need to convince community members that men doing care represent acceptable forms of care work and family.

While there has been some change over the past decade, there is still a recurring thread of suspicion about the proximity of male bodies and children, especially the children of others. As indicated earlier, notable instances of strong community scrutiny can occur in households where single fathers are raising teenage girls, where men enter female-dominated childrearing venues or what one father termed 'estrogen-filled worlds' (Doucet 2006b), and where men are primary caregivers of infants (and concurrently, where women do not take up maternity or parental leave to care for their infants). In spite of the points made here, I would also posit that over time, there has, nevertheless, been some change in the community acceptance of male caregivers.

That is, changing ideologies over time, and the increased presence of fathers in community sites with children are easing at least some of this scrutiny. In my recent work on breadwinning mothers, I have returned to interview twelve individuals that I interviewed over eight years ago. My research program has a longitudinal focus that spans a decade around a small case study of men and women. One example is Richard and Aileen, whom I interviewed three times between 2000 and 2005 and again in 2009. When Richard, a stay-at-home dad, tried to open a home daycare center in 2002, he was told by the local authorities that a daycare facility run by a male would not work in the community. But recently he informed me that things had changed, at least somewhat. He said:

> About three years ago things were getting tight financially. So I decided to try again to open my daycare. I didn't know how they would react to me, but I approached the 'ABC' daycare agency. To my great relief I was greeted with open arms – literally – by a team of open-minded individuals who were excited at the prospect of having a male childcare provider on their team. But one question remained: would a stranger trust a man to care for their child? Well – The answer came quickly. Before all the paperwork and security checks were finalized I already had my first kids! Today my daycare is full with five kids and I have 8 kids on my waiting list who want to come to my daycare specifically. But I am not accepted by all. *Some parents refuse to have a man as childcare provider, and I can respect that. But to many, it is an alternative they favor.*

Where fathers are actively involved in care work, they must work to display not only family forms that 'work', but also that their display of caring and working arrangements with reversed gender roles are acceptable within gendered community norms and judgements.

Conclusions

This chapter has argued that Janet Finch's concept of 'display' can enrich sociological understandings of family forms that challenge traditional or hegemonic gendered assumptions around work and caregiving. Specifically, I developed three key arguments from Finch's seminal article on the display of families.

First, building from Finch's argument that narratives and domestic objects are tools for displaying family, I discussed how narratives, as well as domestic objects, can be used as tools to convey heroic acts towards making families 'work', as well as the display of gendered domestic space, 'happy families' and appropriate masculinities. Second, family forms where men are primary caregivers require an on-going 'process of seeking legitimacy (which) necessarily entails displaying one's chosen family relationships to relevant others and having them accepted' (Finch 2007: 71). Here, I pointed to how particular groups of men must work to display legitimacy, while also managing their displays of care; such groupings include low-income or unemployed fathers, gay fathers, and fathers caring for the children of others.

Finally, drawing from Finch's point (2007: 72) about how it is important 'to think about *degrees of intensity* in the need for display, depending on circumstances', I have argued that the intensity of such displays is less related to change at the level of particular families but more related to social and ideological changes. Nevertheless, these ideological shifts are still lagging behind actual patterns of gendered work and care in most Western countries where processes of globalisation, economic restructuring and neo-liberalism have led to situations where women are primary breadwinners in families and where men, by choice or not, become caregivers of young children. I have also argued that there is a particular intensity, or urgency, to the display of care in households where fathers are caring for infants, where women give up the care of infants and where fathers are moving through child-centred spaces where they may not always be welcome.

Notes

1. With women's average hours increasing, the wage gap is narrowing and the financial contribution of spouses is becoming more equal. However, differences still exist. For example, husbands in dual-earner couples earned on average $1,040 per week in 2008 compared to only $740 for wives (Marshall 2009; Perusse 2003).
2. In 2001 paid parental-leave benefits in Canada were expanded by twenty-five weeks, and, in 2006, Quebec introduced a separate and more generous parental-leave policy with three to five weeks reserved for fathers. Correspondingly, Canadian fathers increased their use of paid parental leave from 3 per cent in 2000 to 33 per cent in 2008, with far more Quebecois fathers – at 82 per cent – taking leave than fathers outside

Quebec at 12 per cent (McKay et al. 2011; Doucet et al. 2009b; Doucet et al. 2010).

3.   While I characterise these fathers as 'groups', I am not implying that they are homogeneous ones. Rather, there are particular combinations of gender, class and sexuality that bring men to the point where they need to manage their displays of family so as to avoid negative community judgements.

4.   I am using 'moral' in the symbolic interactionist sense of the 'shoulds' or 'oughts' of socially acceptable behaviour of men and women (see Finch and Mason 1993).

6
Display Work: Lesbian Parent Couples and Their Families of Origin Negotiating New Kin Relationships

Kathryn Almack

Introduction

This chapter draws upon data from a qualitative study of the family lives of same-sex (female) couples in England who had their first and subsequent children in the context of their current relationship. I examine respondents' accounts about how they negotiate coming out as lesbian parents within their family of origin, and their perspectives on how their families of origin 'come out' (or not) within their own social networks in order to claim new kin relationships with the lesbian parent family. These new forms of 'coming out' resonate with Finch's (2007) notion of 'displaying families' – in which narratives around coming out as lesbian parents display meanings of family and contribute to ways in which these meanings are conveyed, recognised and understood as 'family-like' relationships.

The discussion is set within the context of ongoing debates about the extent and nature of changes to family lives. Contemporary sociological debates about family lives in the Western world have been influenced by the individualisation thesis (Beck and Beck-Gernsheim 1995, 2002; Bauman, 2003; Giddens 1992) which connects wider social changes to 'the staging of everyday life' (Beck and Beck-Gernsheim 2002). A key theme is the erosion of traditional constraints and conventions and the associated portrayal of individuals who are more able to pursue their own choices. This has led to associated questions about the degree to which this individualism is incompatible with commitment and the stability of family life. Families have been depicted as being in 'crisis' (Dennis and Erdos 1993; Murray 1990,

1996) or, alternatively, presented as a reorganisation of ways of living in the context of wider transformations of contemporary society (Giddens 1992). One illustration of the two perspectives is the way in which lesbian parent families have been portrayed as characteristic of 'the triumph of a selfish sexual individualism' over the obligations of the family (Phillips 1998) or, alternatively, as 'prime everyday experimenters' who have 'for some while experienced what is becoming more and more commonplace for heterosexual couples' (Giddens 1992: 135). Empirical work has developed a more nuanced interpretation of family lives by focussing on what is actually going on in personal relationships (Jamieson 1998). Conclusions differ about the extent to which individuals are engaged in 'everyday social experiments' but findings suggest that the parenting of dependent children has a substantial impact upon the pursuit of individualism (Ribbens McCarthy et al. 2003; Smart and Neale 1999). Sociological research has primarily focused on heterosexual families but an increasing number of studies have also addressed the family lives of 'non-heterosexuals' (this includes Dunne 2000; Weeks et al. 2001; Weston 1997).

The notion of display work builds on Morgan's (1996, 1999) concept of 'doing families' which has provided a useful analytical tool to explore the complex realities of family living and 'family practices'. As Finch (2007) acknowledges, display work seeks to contribute further to Morgan's work, suggesting that 'families need to be displayed' as well as 'done' and in doing so, she emphasises the importance of social interactions. This chapter focuses on the interactions involved in negotiating coming out as lesbian parents, and explores the usefulness of Finch's concept of display in understanding the ways in which these negotiations simultaneously form part of familial social interactions and family meanings. In particular, the ways in which social meanings about the 'family-like' nature of one's relationships are conveyed to, understood by, and supported by relevant others. While display work is presented as relevant to all families, she also suggests that the need for display may be greater for those families which move furthest away from ideas of what a 'proper' family looks like.

Coming out and displaying families

The meaning of 'coming out' has shifted over time. In its current usage, it assumes 'a dual sense of claiming a lesbian or gay identity for oneself and communicating that identity to others' (Weston 1997: 44). There have been many anthologies of coming out stories (see Penelope and Wolfe 1989, as an example of this genre) and discussions of coming out within academic literature, with a main focus on the individual processes and consequences of disclosing a lesbian/ gay identity. Within the academic literature, this includes psychological perspectives about the impact of coming out on self-identity and self-worth (D'Augelli and Patterson 1995; Elizur and Ziv 2001), and sociological narratives of the individual who has disclosed his/ her sexual orientation (Armstrong 2002; Plummer 1992; Valentine et al. 2003; Weeks et al. 2001; Yip 2004). Donovan and colleagues (1999) usefully identify the notion of 'layers of outness' which lesbians, gay men and bisexuals continually negotiate and re-negotiate:

> Respondents may be out to themselves and to a sexual partner but to no-one else; to some but not all of their family of origin; to some or all of their work colleagues – so they may be out to an individual colleague but not out at work; they may be out and involved in lesbian, gay and/or bisexual activities but not out to their mother, doctor or neighbours. (1999: 695–6)

The literature on coming out has also predominantly examined issues of individual identity. However, becoming a parent within a same-sex couple adds further layers of 'outness' to be negotiated that, to date, have received relatively little attention (but see Lindsay et al. 2006 and Almack 2007).

Women parenting together: the study

This study was based on in-depth joint and separate interviews with twenty lesbian parent couples in England – a total of sixty interviews. Most respondents (fifteen couples) were recruited to the study by 'word of mouth' through the personal and work networks of friends and colleagues. Out of the forty women interviewed, I only knew one woman personally and made minimal use of any well-defined lesbian networks. The majority of respondents identified as being middle class and were educated to degree level or above. One or both women in each couple were in relatively well-paid employment. Thirty-seven women were white; three were African Caribbean.

Twelve couples lived in urban areas and eight in rural areas across England. Respondents were aged between twenty-eight and forty-seven (most were in their thirties) and had been in their current relationship for an average of ten years.

Criteria for this study included a decision to only interview couples who had had their first (and any subsequent children) within their relationship and whose children were aged six and under (children's ages ranged between a few months and six years old, with a median age of two years). There are many variations of lesbian parent family arrangements, including lesbian stepfamilies (where children had been born into a previous heterosexual or same-sex relationship), lesbians who are lone parents, lesbians with adopted children and those with older children. However, by keeping my sample criteria narrow, I was able to avoid variables of wider social processes at play, such as the dynamics and wider family relationships of 're-constituted' families. Weeks and colleagues (2001), for example, state there were many different dynamics at play in their respondents' accounts of parenting in different situations. Further, interviewing couples whose children were still very young enabled me to access accounts of the first stages of negotiating new terrains of coming out as lesbian parents.

Themes covered (and which I draw upon in this paper) included mapping out social networks as part of the joint interview and each woman's perspective on coming out as part of the separate interviews. All interviews were audio taped and transcribed. Preliminary analysis took the form of identifying themes and inter-relations among themes, while paying close attention to cases which deviated from the normal pattern of the data. I then adopted qualitative techniques of narrative analysis with a focus on gaining an in-depth understanding of participants' experiences within a specific culture and context (Coffey and Atkinson 1996).

Fieldwork for this study was carried out in the United Kingdom in 2000 and 2001, and thus prior to recent developments including the Adoption and Children Act (2002) and the Civil Partnership Act (2004, enacted December 2005). These developments may have some impact on the processes of coming out and of recognising and validating 'families of choice' for lesbian parents and their families of origin. Nevertheless, this study reveals some of the complexities of coming out for the different parties involved which still have relevance within the context of the above legislative changes.

Respondents in my study identify becoming parents as a point at which their own parents (and other members of their families of origin) are potentially called upon to engage more directly with their lesbian identity and/or relationship and to negotiate new family relationships. The child born to the lesbian parent couple may also be a grandchild, a nephew/niece, a cousin. In order to acknowledge the resulting diverse range of biological and social relationships, members within each of the couples' families of origin have to negotiate what these relationships to the lesbian parent family mean. Some respondents had step-parents and three women had adoptive parents – which introduces a further layer of complexity to the biological and social family relationships. Some of this work may involve outward displays of family relationships within their own social networks (which may also require negotiating coming out about the lesbian parent family). It also involves displays of family relationships between lesbian parents, their own parents and other kin such as siblings and their partners.

'We're having a baby': coming out to a family of origin

The overall majority of respondents were out as lesbians to immediate members within their families of origin (parents and siblings) and most had been out in this context for a number of years. For two couples, announcing a pregnancy was the point at which they explicitly came out to their families for the first time. They recognised that having children would make it difficult to continue to conceal their relationship if they wanted to negotiate recognition of their parental and familial status within (and also beyond) their wider kinship networks.

Upon initially coming out, many had received some level of acceptance and support from family members alongside recognition of their relationship, although a significant number experienced ongoing difficult relationships with parents who disapproved of their sexual orientation. Twenty-nine women described their relationships with their parents as close or that they were at least on reasonable terms with their parents. Ten women described having very little if any contact with their parents and one woman's parents had both died.

For about half of the respondents, parental responses to their announcement about having a child were positive and supportive, including responses from parents of women who were pregnant and from parents of women who would not have the biological connection to their grandchild. Marcia, for example, whose partner Jan was pregnant said:

> Yeah, my Mum was great, she responded just as she had when my sister was pregnant. She was just delighted for us and she started knitting stuff for the baby! (Marcia)

Here is an example of 'display work'. Knitting baby clothes may not be a regular routine family practice but it is an activity which forms part of Marcia's mother's repertoire of kin-related activities in her anticipation of the birth of a grandchild. Marcia notes that her mother had previously knit clothes for other grandchildren (Marcia's sister's children). Becoming a grandmother to a child born to Marcia's partner (Jan) falls outside the more conventional notion of grandmotherhood. It is not possible to know whether Marcia's mother's was consciously or intentionally 'displaying' an understanding of family-like relationships here. Importantly it does convey meaning to Marcia, who interprets (and relates) this activity as a meaningful display indicative that her mother accepts that this child will be her grandchild. However this example does also raise questions about the extent to which meanings derived from displays which may or may not be intentional, and the extent to which there is or is not an interactive element to display work. I aim to further consider these issues in further discussion of my data in the following.

Many respondents noted that, although they had had a reasonable response from their parents upon initially coming out and that their parents appeared to accept their current relationship, they nevertheless responded differently to the announcement of the couple having a child together. Jan, Marcia's partner, said:

> When I told my mum I was pregnant she just said 'Well I hope you don't want me to be pleased because I'm not'. (Jan)

This response makes Marcia's mother's 'display of' knitting all the more meaningful in signifying her sense of kin relatedness to Jan and Marcia's child in contrast to the absence of display work undertaken by Jan's mother in anticipating becoming a grandmother.

A significant number of respondents reported that their parents' reactions at this juncture were totally negative, including recollections of parents being 'utterly horrified', 'aghast', 'totally appalled' or responding with 'abhorrence'. It is possible some respondents' parents had not fully accepted their daughters' lesbian identity but were able to at least tolerate this knowledge because they could avoid dealing too directly with their daughters' lesbian identity or their relationships. This becomes harder when their daughter or daughter's partner has a child, especially if they want to acknowledge and develop the biological or social kin relationships to their grandchildren.

For most respondents who had received such inimical responses to their announcements about having a child, their parents' views changed over the course of the pregnancy or following the birth of the child. Jan's mother 'came round' when she spent a week with her daughter and accompanied her and Marcia when Jan had a pregnancy scan:

> My mother was then just on board with it … just totally. But you know … I have had to work at stuff with my Mum, it wasn't just naturally OK. (Jan)

Lauren's mother initially cut off all contact with Lauren and her partner Emma following their announcement about having a baby. However, her actions were not supported by Lauren's father and her grandparents. Lauren notes that her mother is 'quite a forceful character and everybody would usually follow her lead but they couldn't on this'. Lauren's mother relented, agreeing to see Lauren but she 'drew a line at welcoming Emma back into the family':

> Emma only really got back in the picture in the last month or so of my pregnancy and we had to rebuild relationships. But my family were not supportive of us as a couple … it put an enormous strain on us and we ended up splitting up for four months. (Lauren)

The above accounts provide samples of narratives, stories of family which Finch (2007) identifies as an important tool for displaying family and kin relationships. People produce narratives – stories – which they tell to themselves and to others about their family and kin relationships. These form a means through which people both develop and communicate understandings of these relationships. Finch notes that these processes are not guaranteed success and are a 'complex, possibly hazardous business' (2007: 78). Finch further suggests that 'there is a real sense in which relationships do not exist unless they can be displayed successfully' (2007: 79).

The above quote from Lauren also suggests that where a form of display is directed at a particular audience, there is an interactive element to display work and that successful display also requires affirmation. Lauren and Emma's attempts to display their family unit to Lauren's mother were initially unsuccessful. One might say that Lauren's mother responded with her own display – a display which indicates the extent to which she is prepared to acknowledge Lauren and Emma to be as a family unit. Her display involves cutting off contact with the couple and when that display work did not receive an affirmative response from the rest of the family, she then appeared to modify the display to 'drawing a line' at having Emma 'in the picture'. When responses received are not positive or affirming of one's family relationships, the costs can be high. Lauren, for example, notes that it put a significant strain on her relationship with Emma.

One respondent, Rosanna, has not come out to her family – Rosanna lives with her partner Linda who had given birth to their son Dominic, who was 8 months old at the time of the interviews. If a biological mother was not out to her family of origin it would be more likely that her family of origin would still acknowledge her motherhood (perhaps as a single mother) and her child's relationship to them. As a social mother, however, in the absence of display work, Rosanna is not seen as a 'mother' by her family, nor are any kin relationships acknowledged between her family of origin and her son. As Finch notes, the intensity of display work may vary. Rosanna's situation provides an example where there is a greater need to display – in order to facilitate acknowledgement of her family and being a mother where these are not easily recognised.

Rosanna's motherhood is displayed successfully in other parts of her life (for example, Linda's parents recognise her as Dominic's mother and reflect this back, referring to her as 'Dominic's mummy'). With her family, it is not that display has been unsuccessful but that her fear of disapproval or even rejection by her family of origin means she does not even attempt any form of display (to her parents and brothers). This alerts us to the need to pay attention to what can and can not be displayed and also to the layers of display work. Not displaying may be intentional because of the perceived risks involved (the fear of family disapproval or rejection in Rosanna's case) but this also has a cost. By not displaying her family of choice to her parents and brothers, Rosanna is constantly on her guard with them: 'you have to watch what you say all the time which is hard'. However, some of the emotions, risks and costs involved here also go beyond what the concept of display can reveal per se. I reflect more on this point in the conclusion.

Following the birth of their children, several respondents refer to the sending out of birth announcement cards or similar to family members – with some expectation that responses would be made but where these were not forthcoming:

> None of my blood relatives sent me anything in terms of presents, cards, nobody even phoned (when Sara had Adam)...I sent out birth announcement cards to everyone, we got lots of responses of course but none came from my lot. (Ruth)

> When Christina was pregnant I said to my mum and dad, as far as I'm concerned this will be your grandchild, I expect you to treat it just the same as your other grandchildren. In the event I had to chase them up when Grace was born to get any acknowledgment, never mind getting them to come visit! (Judith)

Again, this suggests that there may be degrees of intensity in display work and it outlines circumstances where the need for display becomes more intense as a result of changed family circumstances. For respondents in my study, the birth of a child represents one such instance, a point at which recognition and validation of the familial relationships between the baby and the parents' families of origin are sought. The sending out of birth announcement cards represents an activity imbued with meanings around family and kin. Such cards are commonly sent out to family members (and friends) following the birth of a child and in general one might expect responses in the form of congratulation cards, phone-calls and visits – acknowledging the birth of the child and the new relationships formed (the arrival of a new grandchild, a nephew/niece, a cousin) – reciprocating the display of family relationships. This particular element of display work takes on an additional intensity for lesbian parents in order to establish and define the resulting permutations of family-/kin-like relationships and perhaps especially where the social relationships of grandparent/grandchild, aunt or uncle/niece or nephew and so on are not instantly recognised, or, as Judith puts it, need to be 'chased up'.

Displays of families of choice and of origin

It is evident that many respondents worked hard at commitments to families of origin even when they felt let down or had been disappointed with the lack of familial display work. Their accounts demonstrate a deep commitment to their families of origin – to commitments that matter (Williams 2004) – while, in some cases, it is the older generations who instigate what could be described as an absence of commitment.

Weeks and colleagues (2001) and others such as Weston (1997) have documented emerging narratives of 'families of choice'. These may include relationships based on blood ties but importantly also include relationships based on friendships which become 'family-like' in terms of levels of commitment and support. As noted, such narratives form one way through which people display/give meaning to family relationships.

In my study a few respondents did make reference to relationships that characterised narratives about 'families of choice':

> The meaning of family is very different to the lesbian community than in straight families. To me. you know, my family are my strong friendships around me and not necessarily blood relatives. (Elaine)

> What we've done over the years is establish friendships that have a depth of family to them. Adam is a bit short on blood relatives so we asked our friends Hilda and Bill if they would be grandparents and they've taken on that role brilliantly! (Sara)

Sara went on to describe at some length the kinds of support offered by Hilda and Bill and the activities they engage in. This includes loaning money to Sara and Ruth at times, spending some holidays and Christmases together, having Adam to stay with them. She also observed that as Hilda and Bill are increasingly frail (both in their late eighties) that roles are reversing to some extent with Sara and Ruth carrying out practical tasks for them such as gardening work. This narrative is suggestive of, and displays, what it means to them to be family, doing family-like things. It conveys the meaning that this is a friendship that has endured and has qualities that represent and have become embedded as 'family-like' relationships. These narratives are perhaps made more explicit (in recounting to others the role of Hilda and Bill in their lives) as the contours of their family are not as easily defined or necessarily recognised as family by others.

More commonly however friends were not defined as family by respondents or, in some cases, having children also had the potential to disrupt friendship links previously perceived as 'family-like':

> Friends we thought would be really excited and involved haven't really come up with the goods have they...but to some extent family, well Sally's family, have filled that gap for us. (Hilary)

> Interestingly since we had Grace we've seen less and less of some of our gay friends...they've just kind of backed off. Some of that is probably us not having the energy to sustain contacts and to go out as much but yeah...so that kind of strong network we used to think of like family aren't there in the same way anymore. (Judith)

A number of respondents note similar expectations of friendships developing/continuing, some of which were previously viewed as family-like relationships, after they became parents. However respondents here recount experiences of friends having not 'come up with the goods'. At the juncture of having children, friendships that may once have been regarded as being 'family-like' have been disrupted. To some extent it is possible that people's social networks may change upon becoming parents, particularly if others in one's social network do not have children. Here, however, the corresponding absence of display work required to nurture and develop previously deep friendships akin to family is salient because these relationships may also require more explicit – and ongoing – display work in order to acknowledge and sustain 'family-like' relationships that can not be taken for granted.

Displaying new links to others

In this section I turn to examine respondents' accounts of how their families of origin display their family connections to the lesbian parent family to others in their social networks. The data in this section are based on data relating to display work undertaken by respondents' mothers. Respondents in general spoke in more detail, although not exclusively, about relationships and interactions with their mothers. It is only possible to speculate but perhaps, in part, this reflects gendered responsibilities around kin work (Finch and Mason 1993). Relatively little is known in terms of how families of origin conceal or come out about lesbian relatives within their own networks. Even less is known about the strategies adopted by relatives in acknowledging the lesbian parent family within these same networks in order to 'display' kin relationships to the lesbian parents' children.

Many respondents spoke of ways in which family members had (or had not) engaged in activities that conveyed acceptance and acknowledgement of the family relationships that connect their children to their parents' families of origin. Tools of display – as Finch (2007: 74) notes – can include both direct and indirect acknowledgement of the family-like nature of relationships and different types of 'tools' including the use of narratives and personal and domestic objects. An example of an indirect means of display that Finch (2007: 77) refers to is the display of photographs in people's homes which can convey and reinforce meanings about relationships between the displayer and those featured in the photographs. Photographs were referred to by several respondents as a meaningful illustration of both the level of acceptance of their lesbian parent family by their family of origin, and of the extent to which their family of origin felt comfortable in coming out about the lesbian parent family to others within their own networks.

Sandra and Kate's donor has an input into the lives of their children – he is known as 'Dad' to their sons and has an active involvement in their lives. Kate describes how her mother had selected family photographs to put into frames to display in her front room. Following Kate giving birth to their first son, Kate's mother had chosen photographs that were taken by Sandra of Kate, their donor and son – thus a portrayal of what to all intents and purposes could be a heterosexual family.

I had to sit down with her and say look, you can't leave Sandra out of the picture – I mean literally! (Kate)

In more recent years, since Sandra had their second child, Kate has realised that her mother has put up photographs of just the two boys, none including Kate and Sandra. She observes that her mother has put up photographs of her other grandchildren which do include their parents 'in the picture'. Jacqueline (a non-biological mother) tells a similar account of her mother's selection of photographs. While her mother has some framed family photographs in her front room, photographs of Jacqueline, Joanne and their son Matty are only on display in her mother's bedroom, a private rather than a public space where friends may see them. Kate and Jacqueline both report that their mothers accept their partners and treat their children as grandchildren. Here these grandmothers are also confronted with 'coming out' (or not) to others as part of claiming and displaying these kin relationships to others. However, the extent to which Kate's and Jacqueline's mothers had made conscious decisions about which photographs they put up (and where) is not known. Nor do we know if they were fully aware of what meanings their actions conveyed to their daughters (although Kate's account of conversations with her mother would suggest her mother may have some understanding of how Kate interpreted her choice of photographs).

Ali, who gave birth to Amy, tells a different type of story:

My mum told me about a little struggle within herself about putting a photograph of me with Margaret and Amy up in her sitting room. She teaches piano from home and her sitting room is also the kind of waiting room for parents. Anyway she decided to be completely upfront so, basically, it means she's coming out potentially to all her pupils' parents as the grandmother and mother to do with a gay family. She's actually had some very positive responses and she was saying was she felt proud of herself and is more comfortable now talking about us to anyone. (Ali)

It appears that Ali's mother confronts 'coming out' about her daughter's lesbian parent family in a way that Kate's and Jacqueline's mothers have perhaps avoided. For Ali, both the display of these photographs but also the narrative she re-tells about her mother's account about this display conveys her mother's recognition of her daughter's family which extends to coming out to others 'as the grandmother and mother to do with a gay family'.

To some extent this connects with an issue Tina recalls, from hearing her mother talking to friends and referring to Tina and Deborah as Ryan's two mummies. Tina identifies that this is still unfamiliar territory for her mother:

> When you're gay you grow up predicting conversations and avoiding them or having responses ready and of course my Mum isn't used to all that. I hate to think what terminology she uses but whatever – she does accept us and sees Ryan as her grandson just as much as my brother's kids. (Tina)

Tina is the non-biological mother to Ryan. She notes one example of a 'sticky moment' her mother faces as a situation where friends have made comments such as 'I didn't know Tina was pregnant'. As children grow older, questions and stories about pregnancy (as one example) are focused on with less frequency; it is possible that the boundaries between biological and social relationships may blur over time. As noted earlier, family relationships are fluid, subject to change over time as individuals move through the life course and display work is correspondingly part of these ongoing evolving processes. Elsewhere I have discussed how respondents negotiate social encounters with others as parenthood brought them into contact with new social networks (Almack 2007). I discuss, as Tina notes, ways in which they 'predict' such encounters and have a repertoire of responses at the ready in making choices about how to respond to personal questions about their family. In displaying family narratives, inclusive of the lesbian parent family, members of respondents' families of origin may not be so practiced at dealing with such encounters. However, where grandparents forge ahead regardless, as Tina describes her mother doing, these narratives are perhaps even more meaningful in displays which demonstrate acceptance of the lesbian parent family.

Conclusion

The concept of display resonates with my data in examining the ways in which lesbian couples' relationships with their families of origin were, to varying degrees, disrupted and renegotiated at the juncture of becoming a lesbian parent family. It highlights how, for many respondents in my study, having a child required actively negotiating and demonstrating familial relationships with their families of origin. This includes the working out of new kin relationships between their child and their families of origin, the extent to which these relationships were recognised and validated, and also a consideration of the extent to which family members come out about the lesbian parent family within their own networks. This additionally serves to emphasise 'the continually evolving character of the relationships' (Finch 2007: 69).

The focus on the display work undertaken by respondents in my study is also useful in revealing evidence of respondents' deep commitment to sustaining family and wider kin relationships. The increasing diversity of family forms and corresponding sense of fluidity in contemporary intimate relationships has given rise to concerns about the instability and fragility of family lives, where individuals (and younger generations in particular) are perceived to be putting their own interests first with a corresponding loss of commitment to family relationships. However, my findings add to an increasing body of evidence that suggests people are 'energetic moral actors, embedded in webs of valued personal relationships, working to sustain the commitments that matter to them' (Williams 2004: 41).

Being alert to displays which appear to have not been successful (that is, displays which are not acknowledged or which did not produce the desired response) and instances where there is an absence of display work may be particularly useful. It can highlight some of the everyday experiences that Smart (2007: 133) identifies as 'the issues of living in and with ongoing difficult family relationships'. As Smart discusses, it can be difficult for researchers to 'get at' the 'imperfections of the families we live with' (2007: 137). While these aspects of family lives go beyond what the concept of display can reveal per se, the concept can here be usefully employed as an orientating device to examine what might be going on below the surface of family lives. This is a particularly sensitive endeavour in discussing findings about lesbian parent families. Weeks and colleagues (2001: 8) suggest that non-heterosexual parenting is 'probably the most controversial and contested aspect of families of choice', a statement reflected in the latest British Social Attitudes report (a leading annual social research survey on the British public's changing attitudes towards social, economic, political and moral issues). Findings indicate an increasing tolerance of same-sex relationships but not the same level of acceptance of same-sex parenting (Duncan and Phillips 2008). Stacey and Biblarz (2001) have noted that in this current climate, some researchers have adopted defensive conceptual frameworks but they argue it is important to have a full discussion of the vulnerabilities of same-sex families as well as their strengths.

The concept thus provides a lens through which to identify and describe some important elements within my data. For example, Finch's notion of 'degrees of intensity' is useful. Although display is potentially a feature of all families that becomes more or less intense at different points in time, the concept may hold a particular relevance for situations of uncertainty and for families whose contours are not easily recognised. I have discussed, for example, how respondents' accounts demonstrate that having a child in a lesbian parent family is not a simple question of 'adding in' a new family member but has wider implications for the evolving nature of family relationships. This may be exacerbated by the absence of institutional recognition, although recent legislation such as the Adoption and Children Act, 2002, and the Civil Partnership Act, 2004, may make a difference.

However I also identify areas where the ways in which the concept can be employed require further consideration. Finch (2007) identifies social interactions (direct and indirect) as a central component of display work. This introduces the idea of 'audience' and, while Finch does not ignore this point, there are further questions to be addressed. These include the extent to which external audiences (and whether these are real and/or imagined) are involved in acknowledging and establishing family-like relationships, which raises points about the interactive and multi-layered nature of display work. For example, display work may be open to different interpretations; it may be that the display being made is received differently by the external audience and/or carries meanings not intended by the 'displayer'. In a similar vein, some displays of family-like relationships may be unintentional but nevertheless hold significance to others. There are also choices to be made about what is and is not displayed. Thus, there are questions still to be resolved about the boundaries and use of this concept but it does contribute a new dimension to the ways in which people 'do' family, in particular where the need to delineate the form and character of familial relationships takes on a particular intensity.

Acknowledgements

I am indebted to the women who took part in this study.

Notes

1. Five couples made contact with me through indirect routes – an advertisement placed in a national monthly magazine for lesbian and bisexual women (Diva), and a flyer mailed out by a lesbian parenting network in the South West.
2. In England and Wales, the Adoption and Children Act, 2002, came into effect on 30 December 2005. For the first time, this allowed unmarried couples, including same-sex couples, to apply for joint adoption. The Civil Partnership Act, 2004, came into effect on 5 December 2005. The Act applies in Northern Ireland, Scotland, England and Wales and it allows same-sex couples to make a formal legal commitment to each other by entering into a civil partnership through a statutory civil registration procedure. Same-sex couples who register their relationship then have similar rights and responsibilities to married couples including, for example, the right to survivor's pension benefits. See Merin (2002) for a comparative study of the legal regulation of same-sex partnerships worldwide.

6a
Commentary on Almack's Chapter
Liz Short

The 'display' (or otherwise) of families, and the related issue of facilitating recognition of families, is central to the lives of people in the families of lesbian women, as a burgeoning related body of research and concerted activism around the world attest. The legal, public policy, social and discursive contexts in which lesbian women have families vary across time and place (e.g., see Ryan-Flood 2005; Short 2007a; 2007b). The terrain which lesbian couples who have created families have navigated and negotiated, however, has predominantly been one in which the family-related laws, public policies and discourses have been built on and have promoted a family hierarchy and blue-print of the 'real' or 'ideal' family as having one partnered heterosexual mother and father. As lesbian women 'navigate a landscape' in which lesbian-parented families are often not recognised, understood and/or valued (with associated legal, financial, practical, interpersonal and emotional negative consequences), lesbian mothers "show", "signpost", "mark-out", and give cues about how to relate to them *as* a family (Short 2007a; 2007b). Thus, 'displaying' who the family is, and that the family *is* a family (particularly to those outside what might be regarded as the immediate family), are part of the resources and strategies used to 'navigate' a terrain in which lack of recognition, discrimination and denigration are features.

There are many things lesbian mothers do that 'display' family, such as: calling both mothers mum; having no or infrequent interactions with known donors; organising work so that both mothers spend significant time looking after children; emphasising similarities with other, mostly heterosexual, couples who have conceived

119

with assisted reproduction; and undertaking ceremonies and what-ever (often limited) official means of recognition of family relation-ship and responsibilities are available. However, sometimes family 'display' *is not* a central reason underpinning these actions and instead they are clearly related to gendered notions of (intensive female) parenting and economic imperatives, or are everyday things done in many families. Further, there are many things that lesbian mothers do to 'navigate' the terrain that are not (much or centrally) about 'display' or aspects of simply 'doing family', but that have to do with 'resistance' and maintaining resilience (for example, interpret-ing negative interactions politically rather than personally; inten-tionally associating with other lesbian-parented families and keeping in mind that families created by lesbian parents have particular potential strengths). Whilst 'displaying' the family is often, at least in part, intended to aid recognition of the lesbian-parented family, in a heterosexist context 'display' can lead to problems, and is there-fore sometimes intentionally *not* done. Thus, 'display' is done (or not) in a context and for reasons, and has varying consequences, and is one activity or strategy that people can use to shape their interac-tions, identities, well-being and lives.

Thus, in using the concept of 'display' to illuminate empirical work, researchers need to use and recognise 'display' in contextual-ised ways – both alongside other useful sociological concepts and foci in relation to families, and in terms of keeping in mind the legal, policy and discursive contexts in and about which 'display' is employed (both by researchers and research contributors). In rela-tion to this, Almack suggests (Chapter 6) that legal and policy devel-opments may impact on processes of recognising and validating families, including 'display'. Research is indicating that this is indeed the case. For example, the Australian *Conceiving the Family* project compared the experiences and narratives of lesbian women who lived in Victoria (where women without male partners have been prevented, by legislation, from using fertility services and where non-birth mothers have not been legal parents) with those in parts of Australia where lesbian women *are* able to access fertility services and where two mothers *are both* legally recognised *as* parents. Australia has been a world leader in amending family-related laws to remove gender-based discrimination and to recognise *both* women in families created by female couples *as* legal parents and, therefore, such families *as families*. This has been a hard-won change, and one that "makes the world of difference" and has led to "huge" change to the lives of lesbian mothers and their families. Equitable access to fertility services, and most importantly, legal recognition of two women *as* parents makes planning, negotiating and living in lesbian-parented families very much more "secure" and "comfortable" for all involved. This significant legal change provides a very different landscape and materials and resources, and hence strategies, with which to conduct and convey family life (see Short 2007a; 2007b).

Such research adds significant support to the implication in Finch (2007) and Almack (2007) that those who are further away from the dominant normative lens and model of a family might have more need to 'display' family than others: having official recognition of *being* a family means that people have less need to 'display' as such-obviously, these tools and strategies to 'navigate' such things as invisibility, heterosexism and discrimination are less needed when the context contains less of these. To have both mothers on the birth certificate provides a firm and authoritative marker that the family of a lesbian couple *is* indeed a family and that both mothers *are* indeed parents; provides material with which lesbian-parented families can attest that not only do they 'do' and 'display' family, but that they *are* family; makes the need for 'display' less intense; can make 'displaying' less threatening; and provides excellent and irrefutable material and resources (including documents, narratives and discourses) with which to assert and 'display' family. Resonating with the findings of Almack (Chapter 6), these women's parents were also reported to find this readily understood and authoritative designation of family status of assistance in recognising, stepping into and telling others about the family and themselves as grandparents.

It is hoped that by picking up on some important issues and implications in Almack (Chapter 6) and Finch (2007) this commentary contributes to furthering our understandings of how the concept 'display' can both illuminate research about families and be further developed.

6b
Commentary on Almack's Chapter

Roísín Ryan-Flood

A focus on lesbians who have children after coming out – the so-called 'lesbian baby boom' – is particularly useful in considering the varied dimensions of display work. Lesbians who embark on parenthood within the context of an openly lesbian lifestyle are a relatively new phenomenon. As such, there are less-established scripts regarding their kinship configurations. This is particularly the case for the birth mother's partner, who may be a full parent but is not generally afforded the automatic legal and social validation given to birth mothers. Lesbian parent couples are constantly forced to explain their existence as they grapple with homophobia and heterosexism in wider society that is often unaware or unsupportive of their existence. The process of communicating and asserting their family form therefore requires negotiating hegemonic discourses of 'family'. Finch (2007) notes that display work is relevant to all families, not just unconventional ones. However, new kinds of families find themselves grappling with recognition and affirmation, forcing them to reflexively engage with wider norms of display work. This requires that they become aware of wider family discourses, practices and displays in order to incorporate, reinvent or repudiate them in the context of their own family.

Finch argues that unlike theories of performance and performativity, which are more concerned with individual identities and subjectivities, the concept of display work allows for greater consideration of social context. However, a concern with 'context' in the form of space and place has long been present in human geography approaches. Nonetheless, Finch is correct in highlighting the importance of context for analysing family life more widely. In my research on lesbian parenthood in Sweden, the most common family form consisted of a lesbian couple parenting with a gay man or gay male couple (Ryan-Flood 2005; 2009). Yet Swedish law only recognises two parents, displaying an exclusion of those who create families beyond the heteronormative ideology of two parents. Thus, display work can also take place at the macro level, in the legal regulation of who may or may not be recognised as family and reflect a heteronormative or homophobic bias with corresponding implications for custody, inheritance, social welfare and so on.

In my cross national research on lesbian parents in Sweden and Ireland, I found that they undertook numerous strategies of 'display work' in order to affirm their families. One example of this concerns a Swedish lesbian couple who were parenting with a gay male couple. They conceived two boys together and all four parents were biological parents. Their older son attended a daycare center that had a tradition of putting a sign up on the wall congratulating children on the birth of a new sibling. The sign would include the names of parent(s) and children. When their second son was born to the co-parent of their older son, with a different donor father from his brother, the daycare center was confused about their family relationship. Because the two boys were not genetic siblings, they mistakenly thought that they were not brothers at all. However, the lesbian couple clarified the matter and asked that their new addition be 'displayed' on the wall. The daycare assistants put a sign up that grouped the birth parents of one child on one side and the birth parents of the new baby on the other, as if they were two heterosexual couples. The lesbian parents again clarified so that the two boys' names were in the middle of the sign, with the two lesbian parents paired on one side and the two gay fathers on the other, reflecting the fact that their family consisted of four parents – two mothers, two fathers – and two sons. All four parents felt themselves to be equal parents to both boys. This example indicates the importance of display work in communicating and asserting new family forms. In this instance, display work serves to clarify problematic assumptions, raise awareness and project a positive sense of self-confidence about their family and relationships to one another. This positive assertion of their family form through display work also acted as a protective measure against homophobia – they felt that displaying confidence and openness about their family would encourage others to be aware, promote tolerance and instill a similar self-confidence in their children. It would also prevent children from struggling to communicate their family to other children, parents and teachers who were unfamiliar with lesbian parent families. Thus, display work took on both protective and educative dimensions.

This resonates with Almack's findings that we need to consider 'what can and can not be displayed and also the layers of display work' (Chapter 6). Her work illustrates that this is true both of how lesbian parents communicate their family form to their own parents and wider kin, but also in how families of origin struggle to communicate their daughters' new family form in ways that are inclusive. The lack of familiar narratives about how to present these families to wider networks makes display work by families of origin even more meaningful. Display work here is revealing both of the tensions that this new family form encounters, but also solidarity and support. Almack's innovative analysis allows an engagement with 'display work' in lesbian and gay kinship networks to contribute to wider theories in this field. Previous work on queer kinship tends to assume a dichotomy between 'families of origin' and 'families of choice', where the former is associated with alienation and the latter with supportive relationships (Weeks et al. 2001; Weston 1991). Almack's research on display work challenges this dichotomisation.

Finch's concept complements work in geographies of sexualities that explore spatiality, or in the interactive process whereby space and identity are mutually constituted. Gabb (2005b) and Johnston and Valentine (1995), for example, highlight how homespace becomes an important site for the affirmation of difference for lesbian and gay people. Perhaps display work then can be understood as a means of unpacking dimensions of spatiality – the displays that people make inform the construction of space. It remains important to consider the ways in which context, in the form of intersections of culture, welfare regimes, gender and sexuality, inform these productions of spatiality. Display work may provide a useful tool for exploring these processes.

7
Practices of Display: The Framing and Changing of Internet Gambling Behaviours in Families

Kahryn Hughes and Gill Valentine

Introduction

This chapter will consider the additions and affordances the concept of 'display' (Finch 2007) offers in analyses of inter-relational responses to problematic Internet gambling. It will also seek to develop this concept by considering it in both the domestic and public sphere and by examining the issues which arise when family members are not available for 'display'. Display activities in these analyses are not those directly of the gambling, but relate explicitly to family practices of display, and how a perceived absence of these impacts on familial relationships and, often later, of attempts to renew affected relationships.

This chapter draws on data collected in a study funded by the Economic and Social Research Council (ESRC) and the Responsibility in Gambling Trust (RiGT) to look at the impact of problem Internet gambling on the family. In this study, we proposed the home as a key site to study Internet gambling, not only because it is a space where 'new' groups of gamblers like women, young people, and older people can more easily access such activities via the Internet (Fisher 1993; 1999; Volberg 2000), but also because families themselves are so deeply implicated in pathways into and out of gambling (Abbott 2001; Abbott and Volberg 2000; Abbott et al. 2004a; Ciarrocchi and Reinert 1993; Darbyshire et al. 2001; Kalischuk et al. 2006; Krishnan and Orford 2002; Petry 2006; Wardle et al. 2007). Despite this, much of the literature on the family and problem gambling largely relies on gamblers' own, rather than their family's, accounts. Importantly, there is a dearth of sociological research on how families/family practices may shape opportunities to gamble on the Internet, and how definitions of *problem* Internet gambling are produced within these relationships. There is also a consequent need for discussion on how different intra-familial definitions and understandings of what constitutes problem gambling demand different strategies and practices of management, healing, repair and recovery for different family members.

In presenting some of our analyses we show how problem Internet gambling in the family is defined as such precisely when significant others articulate a need for 'display'. 'Display' therefore becomes a mechanism through which family members can negotiate and renew relationships, hence highlighting the use of display as a constitutive as well as expressive mechanism.

Internet gambling and the family

It was basically...well in my eyes it was like it sounds daft but because I didn't have to make the effort to draw the cash out and go to the bookmakers – which was really a bit of fun really, you know, not in it to make money just to put a pound on here and there – but it spiralled as though it was Monopoly money. ... Because I wasn't seeing cash, or even when I was winning I wasn't getting cash handed back, it was just as though it was toy money. (Dale, first interview, sports betting)

The emergence of the Internet has opened up new spaces of gambling; it is estimated that already there are over 2,300 Internet gambling sites, making this one of the fastest growing forms of betting (Eadington 2004). One such new on-line space is the home, leading some commentators to suggest that on-line gambling in the home is more psychologically enticing than off-line forms of gambling because it offers gamblers *anonymity* (e.g., individuals can bet without the social embarrassment of being seen by others), *accessibility* (e.g., people can gamble any time of the day/night) and (controllable) *interactivity* (therefore making it more tempting than some other forms of gambling) (Griffiths 2001). In connection with these ideas, there has been the suggestion that Internet gambling marks a shift from 'social' to 'asocial' gambling (Fabiansson 2008) through the removal of the gambler from 'sociable' locations or playgrounds in which they can gamble (Abbott et al. 2004a). Further, research with off-line gamblers suggests that those who are more likely to experience problems are people who play on their own, and problem gamblers report that at the height of their addiction it is a solitary activity (Griffiths 2001; Griffiths and Parke 2002).

It is in this shift from gambling to problem gambling that an individualistic focus on the isolated gambler becomes both prevailing and problematic. For every individual with a gambling problem, it is estimated that somewhere between a further five to seventeen other individuals are adversely affected by it (Lesieur 1984, see also Kalischuk et al. 2006). Yet, despite this, Krishnan and Orford (2002) point out that research into the effects of problem gambling on gamblers' families has been limited and has not addressed family coping in detail. Where gambling research has focussed on 'the family' it has commonly done so through the lens of the spousal relationship, in particular, the impact of male problem gamblers' behaviour on their wives. Spouses of problem gamblers often have to live with financial insecurity (i.e., inability to pay the mortgage, bills, and even for food) and the threat of creditors (Bergh and Kuhlhorn 1994; Gaudia 1987; Lorenz and Yaffee 1988). Not surprisingly, they report similar physical and emotional harms as do the gamblers themselves (cf. Lesieur and Rosenthal 1991; Orford 1994; Volberg 1994) including: depressive symptoms (Bergh and Kuhlhorn 1994); feelings of self-blame and emotional stress (Lorenz and Yaffee 1988); and even physical symptoms such as headaches, dizziness, hypertension and breathing difficulties (Lorenz and Yaffee 1988). Indeed, suicide attempts by spouses and partners of problem gamblers are reported to be triple those of the general population (Gaudia 1987; Lorenz and Yaffee 1988).

Despite the evidence of implications of problem gambling for families, much academic work on problem gambling adopts an individualistic model. This is both in terms of data collection, which normally employs surveys or interviews with individual gamblers alone, rather than seeking relational accounts from their significant others, and in terms of its analysis, which commonly focuses on the gamblers' behaviour/experiences largely abstracted from the complexities of their wider social relations. Consequently, there is little evidence about how definitions of problem gambling are constituted through relationships with 'significant others', including those who are not in a marital relationship but whose lives may also be closely interwoven financially or emotionally with a problem gambler; for example, partners who may be living either together or apart, children, siblings, adult parents, carers (for example, of disabled people) or tenants/housemates.

This is perhaps surprising given that transitions from childhood to adulthood in Western societies have become more extended and more complex in the late twentieth and early twenty-first centuries (Furlong and Cartmel 1997). When (often adult) children leave the parental home, the family is still the site through which many of our individual biographies and expectations are routed in adulthood. Consequently, families with their traditional ties of love and care, remain a crucial entity, continuing to play a key part in the intimate lives of most individuals throughout their adulthood even when they are physically distant from each other (Gillies et al. 2001; Ribbens McCarthy et al. 2003; Silva and Smart 1999). Indeed, Finch and Mason (1993) claim that continued commitment to intimacy, sharing resources and maintaining responsibilities for each other (in terms of material, practical and emotional support) remain unremarkable features of everyday family life. Such intimate relations would therefore appear to be particularly pertinent in the context of the emergence of *Internet* gambling more generally because it brings omni-present opportunities to gamble into the home. In this way, Internet gambling is often embedded in day-to-day household life and the emotional functioning of the space of the home, and thus a range of significant others and their practices are deeply implicated in the development, recognition and management of Internet gambling as a problem.

Problem gambling: a brief overview

Problem gambling, both off- and on-line, has in the main been considered particularly within the disciplines of psychology. Much writing within this tradition grapples with discourses of addiction in understanding the compulsion of gambling (Black and Moyer 1998; Clarke et al. 2006; Steel and Blaszczynski 1998; Welte et al. 2001) and sociology, where writers have extended these ways of thinking in 'adding' sociology to these approaches (Bernhard 2007); incorporating epidemiological accounts of vulnerable populations, such as those espoused during recent debates about the building of super casinos (Quinn 2001; Volberg 1994); or more broadly of vulnerable underclasses, where vulnerability is less a consequence of emotional inadequacy and more related to deficits in educational or social opportunity (e.g., Blaszczynski et al. 1999). Currently, support for people seeking help for their gambling is provided by public and voluntary therapeutic agencies (e.g., GamCare, Gamblers Anonymous, Gordon House). Within these broader agencies, however, there is considerable slippage and uncertainty around 'problem' and 'pathological' gambling where the first draws upon psychological models of harm (e.g., to one's life circumstances, to significant others) and the second on bio-medical models of addiction (Berridge 1990; Blaszczyniski and McConaghy 1989; see also Giddens 2006; Hughes 2007; May 2001; Shaffer 1999; Yellowlees and Marks 2005). These uncertainties are reflected in an unresolved question about which social agency or therapeutic treatment is most appropriate for problem gambling. This ambiguity is exacerbated by a lack of rich data on who, when and with whom 'problem' gambling is identified/defined, and fails to address how gamblers move in and out of self-identified problem gambling without formal agency support or help (Abbott et al. 2004b). We suggest this ambiguity is further compounded by a continued focus on 'the gambler' as a conceptual abstraction: a focus on the isolated, individual gambler and the quest to uncover the 'essence' of his or her 'problem' gambling. Viewed thus, a gambling problem is something that gamblers *have* rather than something they *do* or produce and reproduce.

Our approach to understanding the meanings and definitions of problem Internet gambling as produced, in part, within and through particular intra-family relationships, makes a significant departure from much of the existing work on problem gambling as an addiction. We consider there is a need for a shift from 'the gambler' towards a fundamental engagement with the relational character of Internet gambling and, in particular, to explore how and when Internet gambling becomes understood as 'problematic', who decides it is problematic and how, if at all, 'problem' gambling is addressed. In this chapter, we thus adopt a relational approach, drawing on research not only with problem Internet gamblers but also their chosen significant others (who in this study included spouses/partners, children, parents, siblings and in one case a carer), to examine the processes through which problem gambling is first disclosed within, and then managed by, families. Here, we follow Stacey (1990) in using the term 'family' not just to refer to the traditional nuclear model but also to embrace the complex and diverse range of arrangements that characterise contemporary modern Western societies. In doing so, we bring together insights from the social studies of childhood and family studies literatures to further inform research within gambling studies.

Study methods

In order to gather data on the relational characteristics of Internet gambling, we developed a multi-method, longitudinal design for the study that built upon previous web-based research (Holloway and Valentine 2002). First, we devised an on-line scoping survey, links to which were posted on gambling and non-gambling websites, especially gambling discussion boards. The survey of six-hundred-one Internet gamblers explored: the social and demographic characteristics of Internet gamblers, when/where they access Internet gambling sites, types of Internet gambling in which they participate, whether it is a sociable or solitary activity, and how much money they gamble. This served as a recruitment tool for the qualitative stage of the research with *problem* Internet gamblers, and it is on these data that the chapter is based. Two waves of life history interviews were completed with twenty-six self-identified problem Internet gamblers (twenty men, six women). We also conducted one-off, in-depth interviews with those whom we designated for the purposes of this chapter as a significant other, elected and approached by the gambler to capture data concerning processes of meaning formation around 'problem' gambling. Most often the significant other was a partner, with other nominated significant others including a child, sibling, parents and a non-kin personal assistant (n = 69 interviews). Participants were recruited from across the United Kingdom in both rural and urban areas, and with one exception, all the interviewees were white. They were aged from nineteen to fifty-five years old, their occupations ranged from unemployed through to professional, and they engaged in a diverse array of Internet gambling activities including bingo, slots, poker and sports betting (football, rugby, cricket, tennis, golf, horse racing, dogs, etc.). The sample of interviewees included people with a diversity of gambling histories. Some participants have been gambling for years and were still gambling at the end of the research process. Others had gambled intensively for short periods (e.g., six months), losing thousands and in some cases hundreds of thousands of pounds, but no longer gamble. Others still had lost significant amounts of money but this had not resulted in major financial difficulties for them. Nonetheless, they all self-identified as 'problem gamblers'. When the term 'gambler' is employed to describe the interviewees it is used as shorthand for problem Internet gambler.

The time gap between the first and second interviews with the problem Internet gamblers provided real-time accounts of individuals' experiences of Internet gambling, including in some cases individuals' efforts to reduce or stop this activity because of the effects it had, or they feared it may have, on their finances, family and work. The interview schedule for the first interview was developed in conjunction with the questions for the on-line survey and data gathered were subjected to systematic multi-stage qualitative analysis (Baxter and Eyles 1997). This interview process produced twenty-six cases. A case included all data (including notes and recordings of informal conversations where permission was granted, ethnographic field notes and in some cases on-line diary material) on every interaction involved in accessing the problem Internet gamblers. Building on previous research under the ESRC Research Methods Programme (Emmel et al. 2005), analyses involved inter- and cross-case comparison, identifying linkage and divergence with existing survey data (Emmel and Hughes 2009).

Multi-phased trajectories of participation

Our sample of Internet gamblers are a diverse mix of people, playing a range of on-line, and often off-line, games. Nevertheless, a core linking identity for these participants is that of 'problem gambler'. In exploring similarities between participants' narratives of their gambling experiences, participants generated what could be termed as accounts of *multi-phased trajectories of participation*; namely, their movement into and out of Internet gambling practices, and how these are produced within and in turn, productive of, particular relational practices. Without intending to posit an invariant account of 'becoming problem gamblers', it is nevertheless useful to consider participants' explanations of how Internet gambling practices describe trajectories of gambling, moving from phases in which they begin to gamble, 'maintain' their gambling, to problematic compulsion to immersion in gambling, and then for some of our participants, through phases of 'recovery' from problem gambling. In considering these shifts in practice and meaning, we are able to observe the negotiation processes entailed in reworking these practices as problematic within their intimate relationships. Key to our analyses of this meaning formation and negotiation of problem gambling was Finch's work on 'display'. In order to understand the centrality of the importance of display in negotiation processes between gamblers and their significant others, the chapter will outline some core aspects of gambling trajectories as described by the study participants, and will consider how analyses of these core aspects both identify how problem Internet gambling in the family is defined as such precisely when significant others articulate a need for 'display'; and also will consider what contributions to this concept our analyses from this study might be able to offer.

Relational context of internet

Beginning to play: the circumstances

Participants' accounts in our research of how they began participating in Internet gambling identify a configuration of particular circumstances which provide a *relational context* which they identify as amenable to beginning to gamble on-line more purposively and, over time, more intensely. Core similarities in these circumstances include opportunity, time, boredom, and for quite a few participants, an unexpected flush of extra money. One of the commonest motivations for beginning to gamble on the Internet was boredom as a result of too much time alone, boredom within their home and their family relationships, and the desire for something fun they could do with the time they had available. Commonly, participants link together particular times in their relationships where their partner was absent, or they themselves were absent from their home for a time, and that they had enough money to begin playing.

| Interviewer: | So when did you actually start, start this? |
| Charles: | Probably around about April of last year T [wife] moved … T was working quite local to here so she |

was home every day. Round about April of last year she actually moved jobs and moved down to S [*place name*] to work during the week, Monday to Friday, and it made it very difficult for her to get home and everything, so effectively I was here Monday to Friday on my own and was pretty much bored. That just added to the temptation of wishing to gamble as a pastime if you like, to do something and then it just took a grip and just lost all control whatsoever I had on it at all. (Charles, first interview, blackjack, casino)

In effect, participants draw on ideas described elsewhere in the literature about how Internet gambling involves a whole set of *virtual* spaces, relationships, money and forms of engagement and play (see Reith 1999 for a discussion of this); we have many examples of this (e.g., in Dale's reference to the idea of 'Monopoly money' earlier). However, participants' accounts suggest this relates mainly to the sorts of opportunities available on-line, whereas the circumstances and context of their play is profoundly rooted in material practices and relationally bound spaces. In this way, what our participants say challenges the idea of the solitary player or the isolated individual operating independently in a virtual world. Integral to these relational contexts are the processes whereby, when participating in Internet gambling, participants also describe how these practices form part of identity maintenance and constitution (Hughes 2007).

What I do and who I am: identity and living practices

I'm quite arrogant when it comes to my opinion on football or cricket, especially cricket, you know, I think that I know what's going to happen. And often I do a lot of research into it. It's very rare in sports, you know, betting that I will just put money on something, I will just do a lot of research on it. (Jai, first interview, sports betting)

In the context of the relational settings in which Internet gambling became something they *did*, participants also described how their choices of which games or sports on which they gambled reflected the sort of person they *were*. For some, on-line poker provided an opportunity to learn a new game, challenged and excited by its incremental skill levels, enjoying the social character of play, and enjoying the length of time a game might take. For others, the slot machines required no mental agility, but could be played several times a minute, providing immediate results very rapidly. On-line bingo was seen as a sociable form of play, providing opportunities to visit chat rooms, and socialise with other players; and sports betting required knowledge of the field, whether horses, football, and so on. It thus emerged that gambling practices shape and are shaped by identity practices on the part of the gambler and, therefore, become part of who that person is.

Our analyses additionally suggest that gambling practices profoundly shape what we term 'living practices', those practices in which we engage as part of living for, and with, others. Drawing on previous work (Hughes 2007), we argue here that *identity practices* must always be conceived as part of living practices (*I being for the other*, Bauman 1992) so that rather than theoretically engaging at the level of the individual, we must always engage at a relational level of individuals in the plurality and, importantly, individuals in terms of the networks they constitute and the relationships they configure. Practices, as we use the term here, involve more than identity constitution or the production of *momentary identities* (Bauman 1992); they are predicated upon and involve participation and reconfiguration within extended configurations of interrelations, such as those constitutive of family and intimate relationships. Identity constitution and maintenance, therefore, occur beyond the level of the individual, and are simultaneously constrained and productive of the relational configuration in which 'identity migration' (from gambler to non-gambler, for example) occurs. We would add that Bauman's (1992) *I being for the other* is embraced within the concept of living practices which extends this notion of the other to embrace these broader relational configurations. Living practices refer, therefore, to the reproduction of the conditions necessary for ongoing discursive constitution of human selves. In this context, participants' accounts of their Internet gambling practices describe how these change and constrain how they engage in their intimate relationships and, consequently, how their Internet gambling re/shapes these intimate relationships over time.

It is at this point that we now turn to consider Finch's (2007) concept of display. In particular, we are interested in her understanding of how display operates as a mechanism by which such living practices are *recognised* as family practices.

... the meanings of one's actions has to be both conveyed to and understood by relevant others if those actions are to be effective as constituting 'family' practices. (Finch 2007: 66)

In developing this concept, Finch adds that practices of display serve to both identify bonds as family bonds, and further hold these family networks together *as* family networks. Our analyses in this study would further suggest, as Finch goes on to say, that practices of display are used in networking threatened relationships over time and through processes of difficult change and the reworking of meanings of these relationships. Thus, our analyses suggest that not only do practices of display serve to *identify* relationships as family, but also to support the *reworking* of relationships as family relationships (Finch 2007: 72).

This concept of display is both timely and relevant for our analyses in this study. In particular, it has suggested a means by which we might conceptualise and understand particular practices described by our participants in the ongoing management and renegotiation of their intimate relationships required both in *defining* and *understanding* problem Internet gambling, and *managing* the *reworking* of intimate relationships damaged and threatened by the gambling. In other words, practices of display are *constitutive* practices, rather than (as the term might seem to suggest) a form of family aesthetics. It is this strand of Finch's work that we will take forward.

The remainder of this chapter, then, will look at the particular features of participants' narratives as they describe how, when and with whom Internet gambling practices were reformulated as *problem gambling*; how meanings of problem gambling migrate over time as they are reworked within intimate relationships; and how the ongoing management and negotiation of problem gambling require identity renegotiation for the gambler, and also renegotiation of the meanings, possibilities and practices of their intimate relationships. The chapter will illustrate how core to processes of problem identification by significant others is the articulation of the need of practices of 'display' by the gambler; and equally central to processes of 'recovery' both for the gambler and their family relationships.

What is problem gambling?

A key finding from our study is that 'problem gambling' was not identified as any one thing. Whilst several participants and their significant others drew on models of addiction, others refused to do so. For some participants, the key problem as it initially emerged was debt, whereas for others, the main problem was the continued withdrawal of the gambler from 'doing family' things, such as family meals, childcare and so on. Physical withdrawal was often framed within a broad category of not 'being there' emotionally; in other words, failure to engage in practices of family display signified an absence of family engagement.

Where participants drew on discourses of addiction, or described their behaviour as *compulsion to immersion* as described elsewhere in the literature (Quinn 2001; Reith 1999, 2006; Wood and Griffiths 2007), a key feature of the problems arising from this was the gambler's increasing awareness of this as a problem because of the (current/ potential) emotional difficulties it was causing with, and for, their significant others. Despite the emotional problems, and often imminent financial problems, their gambling was causing their significant others, they nevertheless felt compelled to continue gambling.

For a significant number of our participants, *debt* was the main initial problem resulting from Internet gambling, as identified by the gamblers and their significant others. For these participants, their significant others were often aware that they gambled on-line, may have even been aware that at some point this might have resulted in money difficulties, or even have been discussed as a possible personal problem for the gambler between them. However, 'disclosure' as identified by the gambler and their significant others was the point at which the full extent of the debt accrued through gambling and, consequently, the extent to which the gambler had been involved in gambling in terms of time spent on-line, was made known to their significant others (Valentine and Hughes 2010). Prior to disclosure (often forced by withdrawal of credit from financial institutions, or the issuing of legal proceedings against the gambler and his/her family), gamblers often described hiding their gambling by going on-line during times their significant others were asleep or away; withdrawing from family situations and lying about what they were doing; or getting up before the rest of the family awoke. Thus, participants identified their gambling as problematic when they were no longer able to 'hold off' the gambling from shaping their broader relational practices, such as deliberately starting an argument so that the gambler could withdraw from the family. In this context, practices of display featured those of withdrawal; for the gamblers, these had the effect of facilitating a retreat from family and an immersion into their gambling. For their significant others, these and other gambling practices were reframed as not 'being there'.

Not 'being there': an absence of display

For a large section of our participant sample, a key problem was lack of time spent with the family, where the gambler was not 'being there'. We would suggest that in this way our analyses add to the concept of display which is frequently used to describe public display practices as a means by which family identities are constituted and reinforced in broader social networks. Our analyses suggest that these practices are crucially important in maintaining and, often, re-negotiating intra-familial relationships.

For our participants, not 'being there' involved physical withdrawal from family spaces, and continuing absence from family activities. Not only were the gamblers not there as participants in family events, such as going out, socialising with friends, being involved or engaged in what the children or others in the family were doing, but they were *seen* to be absent by close friends and extended family. For example, one participant played for long periods of time, even during dinner parties at her own home, and in a shared holiday with friends, spent much of her time at the Internet café where she could continue to play on-line poker.

Interestingly, in our study we accessed a small number of participants and their significant others where neither party considered the Internet gambling a problem. In these cases, it was precisely the relational location of the Internet gambling within the home that was seen to provide additional controls unavailable in off-line venues. In these cases, *being there* refers also to the co-presence of significant others who represented responsibility for the Internet Gambler; who in turn is seen to have the right to do what they want as long as it does not cause harm to their families. In one case, time away from families is overcome by situating all the computers in one room so the father can gamble whilst his children do their homework. In another case, the Internet gambler gambles on the sofa beside her partner whilst he watches television. In this way, people synchronise their off- and on-line space-time practices, retaining visibility and engagement in off-line relationships whilst simultaneously shaping new opportunities of on-line participation.

'Being there' emerged as a central theme from our significant-other interviews and played out in a number of ways. Across our sample, debt and money problems migrated over time and were reframed as emotional problems for the gambler and their significant others. Even where participants had not accrued debt, disclosure revealed the extent of their compulsion or involvement in Internet gambling and regular spending which partners often resented or condemned. Money spent was reframed as lack of responsibility, wasted opportunity, and indicative of a normative gulf between the Internet gambler and their significant other. Processes of disclosure, therefore, entail reworking meanings and understandings of 'the problem' – not once, or twice, but over long periods of time. Not 'being there' significantly entailed a failure on the part of the gambler to display their presence and integration within their intimate relationships and families. As mentioned previously, these practices do not refer solely to family aesthetics, but are constitutive of particular forms and experiences of intimate and family relationships. For significant others, not being there displayed a shift, at the very least, and often a betrayal, of the gambler's family identity.

Spoiled identities

Crucially, for both gamblers and significant others, the problem of time away from their families emerged in descriptions of how the gamblers' identities (as parents, children, work colleagues) were 'spoiled'. We are indebted here to McIntosh and McKaganey (2000) for their concept of spoiled identities. Here, when attempting to break from, or make sense of, habituation to a particular set of practices such as drug use, drug-users' attempts to reconfigure a non-using identity often involves narrating how their addiction has spoilt part of or all of their identity. In developing the narratives in this research, participants did the same.

> But I mean there were a number of times where, you know, he [*her son*] would come upstairs, he'd want, obviously would have

something on his mind, want to speak to me and all I would do is get cross with him because I'd lost my hand and it was his fault for talking to me. But I'd also seen both of the kids, both Jenny and Graham chucking things at me and I didn't even notice, you know, I was just so kind of focussed on playing poker. (Claire, second interview, poker)

It was not only the gamblers who described their gambling as spoiling a particular identity. For example, one significant other describes how her feelings for her husband underwent a radical change when she found out how much debt he had run up. The debt spoiled his identity as a provider as it threatened their stability as a family and consequently the well-being of their four children. The debt also represented his betrayal of their children: the time he had spent gambling on the Internet whilst supposedly child caring whilst she was at work spoiled his identity as a father, and with the removal of these two core aspects of his role as her partner, she felt towards him as she would towards a fifth child. The loss of trust, the migration of financial problems as something the family had to deal with, to emotional problems as a result of what the gambler had *done* to the family, were common across the transcripts. Shame, betrayal and loss of trust were universal themes in the narratives, and re-shaping intimate and family relationships were the main 'problems' gamblers and their significant others understood themselves to be working to overcome. It is in analysing how participants' gambling practices worked to reconfigure their family relationships that the significance of practices of display, as practices which *demonstrate* and *constitute* particular experiences of family and family forms, for significant others emerged as a central aspect of their meaning formation of problem gambling. It is therefore not surprising that practices of display emerged as central to some of the strategies for recovery as identified by gamblers and their significant others.

Display and recovery

As definitions of 'the problem' were shaped within the family, so too were strategies for recovery. These 'self-correcting' strategies reflected on the capacities and capabilities of families to come to the rescue, both financially and emotionally, of the gambler. These often took the form of loans or outright payments of debts; in some cases partners returned to work. In one case a gambler's parents even returned to work in order to provide financial help (although, clearly, it was not in the capacity of many families to provide this sort of help).

A frequent consequence of the disclosure of debt was that there was a relocation of control over accounts and other forms of money control, such as bankruptcy, signing over power of attorney, and handing over credit cards. Financial control was commonly taken over by the problem gambler's partner, but for those who were single it was either a parent or an adult child who took on this responsibility. Financial support usually worked as boundary setting for the Internet gambler. As others took on financial responsibility they also set the boundaries for opportunities to gamble. Peter describes the way his father assumed financial control of his affairs:

> ...when I went home [to his parents' home following a gambling related suicide attempt], within five days all my debts were consolidated into one payment to my Dad per month, no interest. It's just a massive weight off and all my cards were cut up, all my accounts were closed. The only account I have is the current account with the same bank of which my Dad dines with the manager, you know [laughs]...I told him [his father] the Monday and on the Tuesday morning we were straight down to the solicitors...who he uses all the time and sat in the front of the bloke who he works with all the time, you know, it must have been embarrassing for him. And then my bank manager and then to the doctors, you know. (Peter, second interview, slots/instants)

Family members also commonly took on added responsibility for control of Internet access such as changing passwords, removing modems, being present when the gambler was on-line to check what sites they were accessing. These forms of intervention, surveillance and monitoring share many parallels with the way parents monitor young children's on-line activities (Holloway and Valentine 2002). Significant others were usually the first to research and also initiate any contact with doctors, counsellors or support groups. Some significant others describe establishing surveillance networks with other family members where disclosure had been extended beyond immediate family members. Gamblers were therefore positioned within broader familial networks in which their 'public' behaviour was observed and reported to spouses/parents in ongoing monitoring processes of the extent to which they abstained or engaged in gambling practices. In this way, both gamblers and their significant others describe the gambler's identity as infantilised, and part of recovery processes entailed regaining adult status within their intimate relationships.

What emerges from analyses of these family strategies for managing both the gamblers' expressed inability to control their gambling, and the ongoing (shifting) consequences of the gambling, are the practices of display in which changes in the relationship between the gambler and their significant other are expressed through particular spatial and embodied practices. Significant others describe standing behind the gambler whilst they work on-line, Googling on the Internet or checking their bank accounts as both a form of monitoring the gambler, but also as a form of *display* of altered responsibilities and power differentials between gambler and their spouse/parent. In Peter's example above, his father directly engages in particular relationships through which Peter may gain access to goods or services he requires in his attempts to move beyond problem gambling. In this engagement, his role as father is re-emphasised whilst, simultaneously, Peter (an adult) is repositioned as child, subject to the decisions made by others around him. Whilst these practices suggest negative, possibly punitive, and often controlling actions on the part of significant others, these are often described as temporary, and fundamentally supportive until the gambler recovers from their compulsion to gamble. In other words, they exist to manage their process of *becoming other* than a problem gambler; and, importantly, to support the repair or recovery of their spoiled identity. This repair and recovery from problem gambling, and repair and recovery of their intimate relationships, is both *signified* and *achieved* through particular display practices.

Spoiled identities, betrayal of trust, negotiations around responsibility and reintegration within relational networks, such as the gambler's family, involve *being there* as an ostentatious practice of 'display'. Gamblers in our sample describe re-shaping their spatial practices in order to demonstrate they are no longer gambling, and that they are actively seeking reintegration within particular relationships. These practices include help-seeking, such as attending GamAnon meetings, or other therapeutic venues, particularly where gamblers' compulsion to gamble was understood within discourses of addiction by themselves and significant others. Several participants describe beginning these fora for their partners, in order to signify their commitment to that relationship, rather than attending for themselves. However, in many of these cases, as time progressed, these fora grew increasingly important for the gambler as they engaged in processes of identity formation of non- or ex-gambler.

Crucially, maintenance of processes of identity (re)formation is achieved through reworking living practices within intimate relational contexts. Thus, participants describe displacing longing to gamble by engaging in family practices such as doing more with their children (part of recovering a spoiled parental identity) and doing more domestic work around the house. In addition, many take up new hobbies and pastimes, and engage in reinvigorating previous friendship networks. Thus, these practices of reworking relational identities involve a fundamental shift in visibility for the gambler both within and beyond their families. They become visible for *not* doing something they were doing often invisibly before and, further, become visible in *formal* relational networks such as self-help groups, and with financial organisations. These practices are also infused with emotional meanings which have resonance within the intimate relationships of the gambler, by providing evidence that they are taking control, taking on responsibility, being honest and facing up to things, getting 'better' (including ideas of illness to those of moral recovery), and importantly that these practices demonstrate an absence of addictive behaviour.

We therefore suggest that processes of 'recovery' simultaneously include practices aimed at reworking one's own identity through regaining a 'non-gambler' identity; recovering and repairing spoiled identities within the gambler's intimate relationships; and, reworking intimate relationships with significant others, particularly around dimensions of responsibility, trust and control. Importantly, 'display' is as much of a practice as other practices identified as part of 'doing' family and, as part of this, 'doing' ourselves. Finally, we would suggest that, on the basis of these analyses, that the importance of practices of display in processes of meaning formation and negotiation of definitions of problem gambling, and the processes and recognition of recovery, are integral to process of identification within intimate relations of how and when significant others *require* practices of display.

Conclusion

This chapter has described how practices of display are core to meaning formation and negotiation within intimate and family relationships. Finch's concept has been both useful and timely; in particular enabling us to grapple with a very complex data set. The ideas Finch presents have been extremely useful as they have facilitated an understanding of the formation of 'problems' and 'solutions' in identity and living practices as described by our sample of Internet gamblers and their significant others, which is profoundly relational. These ideas have also enabled us to generate insight into how 'threatened' relationships are reworked over time, in broader social contexts.

These analyses provide additional relevance for more general theorisation of problem gambling, where problem gambling is often reframed within a discourse of addiction and/or as pathological behaviour. Viewed thus, a gambling problem is something that gamblers *have* rather than something they *do*, or produce and reproduce. In understanding how meanings of problem gambling are produced and negotiated within relational processes, both within and beyond families, we become able to explore how self and family identities are produced, maintained and reworked over time. Practices of display have emerged as central to such processes. They are crucial to both intra-familial negotiations in defining what constitutes problem gambling, and integral to the processes and recognition of recovery. In this way, we are able to offer an understanding of multi-phased trajectories of gambling, in which the processes of change and recovery from problem gambling for gamblers must be understood within and productive of their relational contexts; change for the gambler entails change for their significant others. Furthermore, *definitions* of recovery are similarly negotiated within these contexts. Thus, we suggest the ubiquitous focus on the isolated gambler should be widened to incorporate an understanding of how processes of identity (re)formation require relational rather than individualistic understandings. Finally, in this vein, we would suggest that while practices of display are expressive of 'family', and identifying particular relationships as 'family' both within and without these relationships, they are also *constitutive* of particular configurations of family relationships. Thus, display is not only a conceptual category that we can bring to analyses of family and other intimate relationships but is a normative practice identified within families that is core to their textures, meanings and experiences.

Notes

1. Valentine, G. and Hughes, K. *'New Forms of Participation: Problem Internet Gambling and the Role of the Family'*, ESRC (ES/D00067X/1), March 2006–March 2008.
2. All the names included are pseudonyms; other information which could compromise the anonymity of the informants has been amended or removed to protect the disclosure of their identities. All the quotations used are verbatim. Three ellipsis dots indicates that a minor edit has been made to remove repetitions or verbal stumbles in order to enable the quotations to be more readable. Where a more substantive edit has been made, this is marked in the text in square brackets.

8
Displaying Mixedness: Differences and Family Relationships

Jo Haynes and Esther Dermott

In this chapter we argue that the concept of display can be usefully deployed in the study of mixed families as a mechanism for understanding the experiential dynamics of parental differences as relational and processual. It offers a way of highlighting when ethnic or other differences become salient within mixed parentage families without reifying the mixed category in the process. First we will outline the problems with the mixed category as it is operationalised within academic and policy research, and will explore the usefulness of the distinction between nominal and experiential dimensions of social identity for understanding when, and if, such differences matter. The second section will expand on this discussion by critically engaging with the concept of display as a useful adjunct for illuminating when, how and for whom experiential dynamics of difference within mixed parentage families is relevant for conveying the meaning of family. Using examples from existing research we explore how the conceptual apparatus of display can illuminate the experiential dimension of family relationships, identities and practices. Through applying the concept to this material we argue that there remain key aspects to the idea of displaying family around the ideas of intensity and audience that require more elaboration. These aspects focus on whether the imperatives for family display are externally or internally driven. Finally we draw attention to the methodological conundrum of researching mixedness posed by our conclusions and propose a way forward. We therefore provide analytical insights into Finch's concept of display by deploying it to address intransigent issues in the study of mixed parentage families.

Introduction

Mixed families – those in which parents have different ethnic backgrounds – are increasingly important sites of study in their own right and for providing insights into ethnicity and family life. They provide an instructive lens for understanding how differences are constituted in everyday family relationships, identities and practices. This, in turn, contributes to furthering our understanding of how, in Brubaker and colleagues terminology (2006: 302), ethnicity 'happens'. There are, however, significant conceptual concerns relating to the study of mixed families, mixed relationships and mixed identities which are sometimes sidelined in research. One concern of historical note is the assumption that 'mixing' or mixed identities has tended to refer to inter-ethnic relationships between white and black people or their children, respectively. Additionally, this area of research is often driven by political and welfare-oriented policy agendas in order to tackle disadvantage, racism and other social problems that are experienced by some mixed groups or individuals, with a particular focus on white/black mixing. Such research, which often uses 'mixed heritage' or 'mixed race' as a unifying category of analysis, has contributed to the reification of the mixed category as a 'singular ethnic minority group' (Ali 2007). Additionally, wider use of the official mixed categories from the U.K. Census, 2001,[1] has strengthened their existence as though they are straightforward social divisions. With such challenges, there has been a growing acknowledgement of the need for a reassessment of the field and a reconfiguration of how we might approach mixed parentage families or mixed ethnic individuals without overlooking the everyday experiences of people in mixed families or relationships, or those who claim a mixed identity, by shoe-horning them into an 'objective' category for analytical purposes; by contributing to the further creation of essentialised social categories in the process; and finally by expanding the concept of mixing to incorporate other social differences (such as nationality and religion) that interact with ethnicity in specific and meaningful ways (see for example, Ali 2007; Caballero et al. 2008).

Before briefly tracing some of the pertinent historical steps in the conceptualisation and study of mixing, it is customary to explain the particular terminology to be used. Following some of the most recent research in the area (Caballero et al. 2008) the terms mixing, mixed and mixedness will be used throughout. 'Mixing' enables there to be an emphasis on the phenomenon as a relational and dynamic process for the benefit of understanding how people experience or 'do' family. 'Mixed' is officially in use within the U.K. Census, but it can be used with or without any further specific categorical references as a descriptor of families, relationships and identities, regardless of the specificities of the 'mix'. 'Mixedness' is used to signal the object of study more broadly, encapsulating mixed individuals, mixing between groups and mixed parentage. Finally, we specify where necessary whether we are referring to specific ethnonational dimensions of social difference in mixing.

Trajectory of mixed ethnicity

The study of mixedness has particular historical origins but these are problematic for studying mixedness in the United Kingdom today. Research and debate about mixed identities have, historically, focussed on and been framed by the racial mixing of black and white people. The recent recognition that there are many more types of mixing (Sims 2007) necessarily expands and complicates the idea of what mixedness constitutes.

Academic interest in this subject developed in the United States in response to a legacy of anxiety about miscegenation – the state of Virginia, for instance, refused to acknowledge the legality of interracial marriage until as late as 1967. This anxiety stemmed from the perceived threat posed to the white population by those who transgressed racialised boundaries through cohabitation, sexual relations or marriage, and any offspring of these sexual unions (Song 2003). Traditional conceptualisations of mixedness were not only shaped by the black/white racial binary but also by fear and disapprobation, and as such, problematised mixed individuals from the outset by typecasting them as 'marginal men (*sic*)' (Stonequist 1937) or referring to them as 'half castes'. Pathological conceptualisations of mixing and mixed individuals are now less common, but the black/white racial focus continues to shape commonsense perceptions and until recently, dominated academic research. Within contemporary media and public institutions two types of discourse are currently evident: a celebratory discourse, where mixed people are conceptualised as 'exotic' or as having 'the best of both worlds', alongside the traditional discourse that views mixing as problematic and difficult (Ali 2007), albeit one that often situates the problem with wider society as opposed to individuals.

In the United Kingdom, research interest in mixedness has focussed principally on children of mixed black/white parentage, that is, individuals who define or potentially could be defined as mixed race, rather than mixed partnerships per se. This focus was stimulated by an acknowledgement of the racism faced by people of mixed black/white heritage and a concern that, on measures of social welfare and educational achievement, this mixed group fares badly (Barn 1999; Haynes et al. 2006). Research agendas that have prioritised tackling disadvantage experienced by ethnic minority groups have also begun to include those of mixed ethnicity. In light of both this historical problematisation of mixed individuals and the on-going racism discussed above, research carried out with children of mixed parentage has tended to focus on identities and identity formation in order to, for example, challenge their 'invisibility' in policy frameworks which typically assume 'monoracial' identities (for example, Tikly et al. 2004). In both the United States and the United Kingdom, therefore, it has often been political concerns that have led to an interest in mixed race/ethnicity and policy objectives that have been at the forefront of discussions.

Mapping mixedness

The category of 'mixed ethnicity' is becoming more established within official discourses which, in turn, allows for greater identification as mixed. This is exemplified by the inclusion of mixed ethnic categories in the 2001 U.K. Census.[2] The inclusion of the 'mixed' categories within the U.K. Census made it possible to reliably enumerate this group for the first time; in 2001, 670,000 people in the United Kingdom reported having a mixed ethnic identity (Bradford 2006). It was predicted that this figure would have risen by 40 per cent by 2010 (Song 2007) and it is expected that the mixed group in the United Kingdom will continue to rise even further. This is partly because of the young age profile of the mixed ethnic group – 9 per cent of children are living in families with mixed or multiple heritages (Platt 2009) – and partly because of increasing levels of mixed ethnic unions (Feng et al. 2008), especially from second- and third-generation immigrants to the United Kingdom. There is also the suggestion of a growing 'mixed ethnic community', indicated by the establishment of organisations in the United Kingdom such as 'Intermix' and 'People in Harmony' and the increased media focus on mixed ethnicity. It is interesting to note that significantly more people defined themselves as having 'mixed' ethnic backgrounds in the 2001 U.K. Census (when this category was introduced) than had written in a description of a mixed ethnic background under the 'Other' category in the 1991 census (Bradford 2006).

The increasing numbers of people identifying as mixed and the growing awareness of 'mixed ethnicity' as a valid category with which to identify has been accompanied by a recognition of a wider range of 'mixing', a recognition that mixed ethnicity extends beyond the category of mixed black/white. The four official mixed ethnic categories, as included in the 2001 U.K. Census and, thus, are contributing to current understanding of mixing and mixedness in the United Kingdom, are Mixed White/Black Caribbean, Mixed White/African, Mixed White/Asian and Mixed/Other (see Bradford 2006; Owen 2007 for a fuller discussion of these categories). The 'unofficial' conceptualisation of mixedness however, has now expanded even further to recognise 'mixing' that is not based only on ethnic/racial difference, but includes variations within broader categories and draws attention to religious, linguistic and national differences that are experienced as pertinent to conceptions of identity. For example, recent empirical research by Caballero and colleagues (2008) incorporated types of mixed parenting that are not reflected by the official mixed census categories, including differences based on religion and faith, as well as ethnicity and race. Expanding the mixed category perhaps better reflects the numerous ways in which mixing goes on, but at the same time makes the label 'mixed' a much more confusing one than has hitherto been acknowledged.

Jenkins (1994) reminds us that social identity, regardless of whether or not an ethnic dimension is being referenced, is made up of nominal and virtual dimensions. The 'nominal' dimension captures the name of particular categorisations, for example, British, Brazilian and Buddhist. However, when examining mixed identities some but not all nominal categorisations may come to the fore – an individual may choose to emphasise his or her ethno-national background by identifying as White Irish or his or her national and religious background by identifying a British Muslim. Further, these categories are not of the same order or are they necessarily mutually exclusive. A recent study by Aspinall and colleagues (2008: 22) found that the young mixed people they interviewed drew on a wide range of nominal categories, including combining racial/pan-ethnic terms (for example, black), ethnic terms (such as Somali) and national identity/group terms (for example, English) within the same description.

A further issue is that nominal categories themselves are uninter-rogated and differences within them are rarely discussed. For example, the category 'White' is often assumed to be homogeneous and internal ethno-national differences are overlooked. As dis-cussed above, the mixed ethnicity options in the U.K. Census do not offer any ethnic differences within the White category. The current formation of the Mixed Ethnic category highlights that lit-tle consideration of mixed majoritarian ethnicities has emerged: an individual with parents from (white) French and (white) Irish back-grounds is within current orthodoxy on mixedness unlikely to warrant much attention. While there is of course a need to recog-nise that certain minority ethnic dimensions are dominant in shaping relative disadvantage and experiences of racism, the impor-tant point being made here is that this absence results in a signifi-cant gap in conceptualisations and understanding of what constitutes mixing per se.

Tracing the development of the idea of mixedness highlights that most of what we know has been determined by a narrow range of mixings. This is attributable to the historical black/white focus, the justifiable aim of countering racism and disadvantage, the limited way in which mixedness is officially recognised, the prioritisation of particular types of nominal categorisation and the neglect of inter-nal variation within some nominal categories. Research to date has successfully challenged ideas of monoracial identity and broadened understandings of mixed ethnicity. However, sometimes it has unwittingly promoted the existence of discrete mixed groups which has served to reify certain kinds of ethno-national-racial groupings as constituting mixedness.

All of this points to the importance of increased recognition of diverse and complicated ways in which nominal categories can be invoked. However, mixedness becomes confusing once you move away from relatively straightforward categorisations and open it up to acknowledge all potential combinations of nominal categories. Survey data have often failed to capture this complexity. It has been acknowledged, for instance, that the 'Mixed/Other' category in the census, which encompasses many diverse identities including mixed white ethnic identities, is 'difficult to conceptualise' (Bradford 2006) despite its significant size. This is partly due to the wide heterogeneity within the Mixed/Other category and also because written responses in this category provide incomplete data about the mixed background (e.g., half-Chinese) (Bradford 2006).

Furthermore, a recognition that different ethnic, national and religious backgrounds can form numerous combinations can also undermine the category 'Mixed' to the point where it becomes meaningless for the purposes of analysis. In an era where it is understood that there are multiple dimensions to social identity, it would be hard to deny almost any claim of mixedness. But some people who seem to fit mixedness on the basis of certain combinations of nominal categories do not identify as mixed. Further, some people do not use any ethno-national-racial nominal categories to describe their dominant social identity and instead may highlight something else such as parental role or occupation as more salient. Research by Aspinall and colleagues which explored how young mixed race adults perceived the variety of identity options available to them supports this view, highlighting that the majority of their respondents 'did not experience their *mixedness* as being that central to their day to day lives' and instead, for most respondents, what mattered more were 'their families, their studies, and their wider interests' (2008: 6, emphasis in original).

The virtual (Jenkins 1994) or experiential dimension of social identity, to use Brubaker and colleagues' terminology (2006), refers to the demonstration of meaning or, in other words, the content of a nominal category. The distinction between nominal and experiential/virtual creates the opportunity to distinguish between mixed parentage as a description based on the fact of nominally different parental backgrounds and parenting that involves interactions that are experienced as mixed; where parental differences become salient. A useful way of approaching this distinction is that, as articulated by Brubaker and colleagues (2006: 314):

> As a nominal phenomenon, 'mixedness' is a continuous and stable property of a relationship or an interaction; as an experiential phenomenon, it is episodic and intermittent. In the nominal sense, an interaction or a relationship *is* mixed; in the experiential sense, it *becomes* mixed – in the sense that it comes to be *experienced* as mixed – at particular moments.

Thus, as illustrated by Brubaker and co-workers' example (2006: 301) in research focused on Hungarians living in a small Transylvanian town, although Hungarians and Romanians interact in a wide range of social relationships, it does not follow that these interactions are experienced as inter-ethnic mixing; they are often interacting as parents, friends, colleagues or lovers in a manner where, much of the time, ethnicity does not matter. In other words, these interactions are nominally inter-ethnic, they are not *experientially* ethnic.

This point is important when looking at personal relationships. There is still little understanding about how, when and for whom, dimensions of social identity become *experientially* salient within family practices and relationships. Mixed parentage research has largely focused on children's 'mixed' identity alongside an interest in parental – often mothers' – perspectives and involvement in their identity formation as a way of countering pejorative racialised conceptualisations of mixed identities as confused or 'marginal'. In contrast, there is little research which focuses on the process of parental negotiation in mixed families. Therefore, instead of the starting point for understanding mixedness being driven by a focus on certain nominal categorisations, we should aim for an understanding of mixedness that allows for a recognition of how and when and for whom, within family life, mixing becomes experientially significant. The salient question that should drive future research on mixed parentage could then be: How is mixing subjectively *experienced* as socially significant? In this way, those mixings that are critically significant will be identifiable but not at the expense of reifying mixed categories. By focusing on experiential aspects of interactions in mixed parentage research, we can identify how parental differences shape family identities, relationships and practices without invoking nominal and essentialised categories as explanatory tools.

Displaying mixedness

So far we have argued that there is a need to move beyond approaches to mixedness based on the prioritisation of certain nominal mixed categories towards an understanding of mixedness in experiential terms. We suggest in this section that the concept of display can help us in this task and draw on two particular elements raised by Finch, namely 'degrees of intensity' and the 'audience' for display. In the discussion about audience we include the issue of control which is not explicitly addressed by Finch. Using examples from existing research on family life we highlight how display can illuminate our understanding of mixedness but also explore some aspects of display that, although significant, are currently less well developed.

Intensity: when display matters

Finch suggests that rather than display being suitable for the interpretation and exploration of specific family 'types', it is more useful to consider '*degrees of intensity* in the need for display, depending on circumstances [...] where the need for display becomes more intense' (Finch 2007: 72; emphasis in original). This aspect of display is helpful in two regards. It suggests a focus on moments when there is a requirement or a desire to display family in some form or perhaps more accurately when there is a cultural expectation that specific family circumstances will be displayed through certain actions; Kehily and Thomson's discussion of pregnancy (this volume, Chapter 4) provides an example of one point in the life course when this demand is prevalent. 'Degrees of intensity' also suggests that circumstances will determine the extent to which display is required; Almack's research on lesbian parenting families (this volume, Chapter 6) highlights how families whose circumstances differ from the hegemonic form may display family as an overt strategy. Therefore, display can draw attention to when ideas of family are created and recreated.

More specifically, in relation to mixed families this is a valuable intervention as it allows us to move away from specific categories of mixedness that are often expected to be a priori worthy of study. Instead we can identify when different ethnicities, religions, nationalities, and so on become salient or require negotiation. Intensity of display therefore enables us to observe when social identities are experiential. As an example of a 'moment' when there is a requirement to display, decisions over wedding arrangements might prompt debate about religious identity: How does a couple with different religious backgrounds or an individual who has more than one religious heritage acknowledge both or decide to prioritise? Nationality may be most clearly exposed at a different moment, for example, expectations about childcare practices that are revealed once children are born.

Thinking about the intensity of display makes it possible to recognise that different forms of mixing have greater or lesser social significance, and that this is determined by social location. For instance, mixed families may change how they assert and present themselves as a family if the ethnic, religious or class composition of their residential area changes either through their own geographical relocation or the introduction of new individuals or groups in their local area. A mixed ethnicity child of White/Black Caribbean descent who lives in a single-parent household with their white mother and in a community setting that is predominantly white is likely to have to consider ways to display family membership in order to be socially recognised in a way that a child of similar racial heritage who lives with two parents in an ethnically diverse community will not.

A research project conducted by Edwards and colleagues (2006) on sibling identities and relationships demonstrates both these elements of intensity; both circumstances which mean display is necessary and a moment when display is possible. Edwards and co-workers quote from interviews with two siblings discussing how they stand up for each other when they experience bullying: 'Once when Jessie, yeah, this boy in her class kept kicking her and Mark, yeah, said, "Leave my sister alone"' (2006: 71). This can be read as a display of family, made through taking care of a sibling who is in some way under threat by outsiders. As such it highlights a moment in time when being a sibling becomes relevant. Additionally, the researchers' raise the possibility that the particular family circumstances of this group of siblings – being of mixed ethnicity and living in a predominantly white area – may have led to bullying on racist grounds. This incident of display also emphasises that social positioning will lead some families and family members into displaying practices as family more overtly and frequently than others.

Audience: controlling displays

The concept of display also draws attention to who is involved – as actors and audience – in signifying family, as Finch emphasises that it is social interaction which is central to the idea of display. Our position is that it is the audience element, in that display must be done by social actors to an audience, which provides a necessary emphasis. In terms of what is of additional value to previous discussions of how the sociology of family should be approached, Finch's concept of display provides a particularly useful emphasis on *who matters* when it comes to experiencing and negotiating difference within families. As is evident from existing research on mixed parentage families there are multiple audiences to whom display can be directed. We know that specific audiences – whether individuals, groups or institutions – are critical to the shape and meaning that family practices, identities and relationships take. In mixed families, key people such as parents, grandparents, friends or peer groups and institutions such as schools are significant for displaying mixedness.

We propose that the idea of the future audience is important in thinking about who matters for display: the audience does not necessarily have to be conceived as immediately present in the family's social milieu. It may be the case that aspects of the meaning of family displayed are for 'future audiences' or the imagined audience constituted by individual social actors or institutions. We know that ideas about what constitutes a particular family role varies depending upon the audience; for example, in relation to the idea of 'good fatherhood', equal responsibility may be emphasised to a partner, open communication and friendship may be prioritised when interacting directly with a child, while ideas of breadwinning persist as culturally important (Dermott 2008). Specifically, in relation to some mixed parentage families, critical decisions are made about alternatives that have long-term display implications; decisions about religion, language or children's names suggest an on-going display of the family identity developed within a particular social context, rather than something that can be redefined or created on a moment-by-moment basis. In Brubaker and colleagues' aforementioned research, Romanian and Hungarian nominally mixed marriages or partnerships were experienced as mixed often when there were specific choices to be made between 'ethnically marked alternatives – marriage ceremonies, children's names, religious practices, language use, and schooling', described as 'ways that make ethnicity happen (Brubaker et al. 2006: 303). We can see that children's names, religious practices and language use have on-going display implications, even though the audience of such displays may not yet be known. As a mixed family the longer term implications for selecting a Romanian or Hungarian language school is viewed as a choice that is 'understood to have enduring and widely ramifying consequences, not least for the child's eventual identification as Romanian or Hungarian' (2006: 313). Thus this choice of meaning for the family, determined in part by school choice, is a continual display of family. The process of naming children provided a moment for parents to convey a particular idea of family which has longer term implications, by either foregoing both Hungarian and Romanian names in favour of either international names (not Hungarian or Romanian) or using translatable names (that have equivalents in both Hungarian and Romanian). The names selected within mixed families constitute an on-going idea of the family – this can be viewed as either conveying a homogeneous family identity reflecting one aspect of the parents' backgrounds (e.g., ethno-national identity) or an alternative way of naming that does not reflect either parent's background.

A related concern is the role of the audience in determining display, that is, who has control. Implicitly the impression given in Finch's discussion is that it is actions performed and decisions taken by individual family members or groups which constitute displays of family and therefore the idea of display suggests a significant degree of agency and control by those individuals who are engaged in family practices. While display may be a considered meaning-making activity by family members, emphasising this element downplays the way in which cultural expectations about family and familial relationships are formed by members of society in general. In relation to the example from Edwards and colleagues (2006) (quoted previously), there is an active decision by the siblings to behave towards each other in a protective way, but this is a decision which is provoked by external events.

The necessity to engage in particular forms of display is in response to wider societal expectations and, even more strongly than this, displays of families are frequently produced by outsiders and may be imposed on family members. An exploration of black and minority ethnic (BME) children in care and their placement outcomes by Selwyn and colleagues (2008) highlights this issue. Interviews with social workers and an extensive examination of case notes revealed that ethnicity was considered important when finding long-term foster care or adoption in order that children were brought up in a household that 'matched' their family of origin, following from a professional belief that this would reduce the likelihood of mental health difficulties in the future. However, the display of mixed ethnicity was not one that was necessarily actively constructed by any of the family members involved (child, parents or extended family). Here instead the power to control family membership lay with social workers and adoption panels and their decision-making processes, which engaged with the views of actual families to a greater or lesser degree. What was really striking about the researchers' findings was the way in which the child's family's current circumstances could be overruled by the social workers' views on what should 'count' in terms of ethnicity, so that a mixed ethnicity child who had been brought up by a single white mother, whose father's ethnicity was unknown and who had been fostered by a white couple could be categorised as 'black'. This instance highlights, with a relatively extreme example, how displays of family need not be based on the experience of family relationships and identities: this seems quite distinct from the forms of display highlighted by Finch where the focus is much more on the creation of familial identity through forms of display in events that are commonplace to many families.

The above examples highlight the importance of acknowledging wider social and political implications of meanings attached to family and thus how the concept of display can be usefully applied provided that the complex aspects of audience and degrees of intensity are properly taken into account.

Implications for future research and concluding discussion

If an aim of research on understanding mixed families is, as we believe it should be, evaluating whether and how mixedness becomes relevant in everyday life, this sets up a methodological problem of how research can be conducted. In the past, research on mixing has focused on particular forms of (usually ethnic) mixing and has targeted groups who fit certain nominal categories or has concentrated on individuals who self-identify as mixed. While this research has been valuable and has broadened the understanding of what counts as 'mixed', it still presupposes that 'mixed' is a significant category of analysis. Because our starting point is to argue that many people may recognise themselves as mixed or being in a mixed relationship only at 'signal moments', mixed need not be assumed to be a constant salient identity and indeed, depending upon the form of mixing involved, may remain irrelevant or even unrecognised. This position allows us to focus both on moments when individuals may actively choose to display their mixed family and when display is forced on them by external observers. However, it is less easy to see how these can be captured in research encounters. One approach is to focus on periods of transition and significant events in families, that have been demonstrated as of interest by previous research, rather than particular groups, and simply being aware of the possibility that mixing and the negotiation of a mixed identity could be an emergent theme. Events could include both traditional rites of passage – weddings, births and funerals – as well as 'newer' rites of passage such as going to university, cohabitation and home buying. This approach would mean downgrading the a priori importance of mixedness but being more alert to the variety of mixing and where it may emerge. It is in the data collection stages that the experiential aspect of mixing is often compromised by leading questions or the imposition of analytical categories which this approach would also avoid. In practice, we would suggest that the revisiting of archived qualitative research on family relationships, including studies that were not themselves especially focused on the negotiation of mixedness, could be useful.

The understanding of contemporary families has benefited by scholarship that explores how families are defined and experienced through ordinary practices, identities and relationships (Morgan 1996); in other words, a move from 'being' to 'doing' family. Finch's concept of display has expanded on Morgan's concept of *doing* family by emphasising how practices need to be conveyed and understood as family by others. We have taken up the invitation from Finch to both refine and use her concept of display by providing an account of how display can be applied to mixed parentage families. In refining the concept we have highlighted two main issues.

The first issue relates to Finch's 'degrees of intensity' which marks out when display becomes significant. Following on from her idea of 'moments' of significance, we have highlighted how these moments need not relate only to transitions between family forms (like divorce) or be other commonly recognised markers of transformation in family status (like leaving home) but can arise from a much wider range of social interactions. For example, a change in geographical location may lead to siblings displaying family as a response to racism. Similar to the way in which Morgan (1996) describes how different practices can be described as *family* practices depending upon the focus of the research, transformations and transitions that are not explicitly to do with family can still themselves prompt displays of family.

The second issue concerns the audiences for display. The audiences are not passive consumers of display but are actively engaged in the process of creating the meaning of family. We identify three ways in which this is manifest. The first emphasises how external definitions of family can be imposed on family members, such as rulings by official bodies about which aspects of family culture are most important. The second highlights the perhaps taken-for-granted point that audiences can inadvertently require familial displays that would not otherwise take place. Finally, responses of audiences cannot necessarily be anticipated because they are not always immediate, thus some practices necessarily require the anticipation of future perceptions of social identity. We have demonstrated the further analytic potential of the concept of display and how empirically it can be put to good use. This also provides a way forward for thinking about how the problems within the study of mixedness are to be overcome, through emphasising the experiential relevance of mixing, both within family research and more widely.

Notes

1. These categories are Mixed: White and Black Caribbean, Mixed: White and Black African, Mixed: White and Asian, and Mixed: Other.
2. Since 2000 in the U.S. Census, instead of providing a Mixed category, the Census form allowed multiple racial categories to be selected in order to measure multiraciality.

9
'Family Hold Back': Displaying Families in the Single-Location Home/Workplace

Julie Seymour

Introduction

This chapter, in keeping with the overall aim of this volume, takes up Finch's invitation to assess and develop the new concept of 'displaying families' (Finch 2007). It aims particularly, as proposed in the original article, to use empirical data to develop and re-examine the concept (Finch 2007: 73) and to open up further questions for discussion. Displaying families was presented as both an empirical activity and an analytic concept, and this chapter will initially focus on the former to allow the development of the latter. The chapter will examine the situation of families who are living in the workplace to interrogate the utility of the concept in arenas where public/private or commercial/domestic contexts become conflated. It will draw on my research on families running hotels, pubs and boarding houses in the United Kingdom (Seymour 2005; 2007), but also reference other studies of such situations in non-U.K. settings and different cultural traditions (Lashley et al. 2007; Lynch et al. 2009a) to consider the international applicability of the new concept.

The substantive area of 'home-located production' (Felstead and Jewson 2000) allows the consideration of the concept of displaying families as one dimension of those practices/actions which make up multi-purpose social interactions. Using data from studies of the single-location home/workplace highlight occasions when displaying family activities occur alongside other practices; in this case, those of a commercial hospitality business. Here, activities may have a dual purpose, relating to both the family and the business, or may consist of publically witnessed family practices within a business environment. As a result, displaying families in this context becomes a complex mix of presentation and reticence – the family has to be highly visible but not publicly privileged over the guests.

In Finch's original article the activity of displaying family appears to have a generally positive interpretation. Displays are interpreted as revealing the positive nature of family relationships and the fact that 'they work' (2007: 70). This chapter will use research on families in businesses to problematise whether displaying family is an inherently positive concept and, if not, to explore its less positive/negative aspects. Throughout the chapter, the key issues raised in Finch's article of variable degrees of intensity and effectiveness/legitimacy will be discussed.

The empirical research

Many of the examples used in this chapter will draw upon my own research into people bringing up their families in U.K. hotels, public houses and boarding houses. I will also show where the issues raised by this empirical data resonate with those highlighted by other international studies of family businesses (Getz et al. 2004) and, more specifically, those settings which in tourism, business and hospitality studies are called the 'commercial home' (Lynch 2005: 534–5). Here the public, as guests, share dwellings, the same plot of land, or in the case of Jennings (2009) mobile boats, which also home to those running the business. The defining feature of the studies outlined here is they contest the frequently made assumption (Christensen et al. 2000) that work and home occur in different locations.

These international references are pertinent in three ways. First, in relation to the substantive topic itself, the range of studies from across the world confirm 'the global nature of the phenomenon' (Lynch et al. 2009a: xvi). Research on hospitality is both multi- and inter-disciplinary (Lashley et al. 2007; Lynch et al. 2009b: 21). For example, Sloane-White (2009) has examined the cultural and religious understandings of hospitality among Malay Muslims. Other researchers have examined the issues that can arise in commercial homes 'when cultural traditions have been misunderstood or are in conflict' (Benmore 2009: 124; Selwyn 2000).

Second, these studies suggest that the topic has a more general application to the social sciences. As tourism management and

hospitality studies have developed an increased focus on social interactions perspectives, they suggest that 'the commercial home
becomes a space that encapsulates a microcosm of the social world'
(Lynch et al. 2009c: 218). Hence, 'academics from a number of fields
have increasingly looked to these traditional approaches to hospitality as a way of better informing the study of the contemporary world'
(Lynch et al. 2009a: xiv). Finally, reference to these works will allow
the concept of displaying families, although emanating from the
U.K. literature, to be seen as having international application.

To place my own empirical data in context I will provide further
details about my research on 'family practices' in hospitality establishments which are both homes and businesses, such as family-run hotels,
public houses and boarding houses. These somewhat atypical settings
constituted a complex mix of public and private arenas and hence provided a variety of audiences for the family displays which were undertaken. This included family members (both those who lived on and off
the premises), guests and staff. Thus the initial scope of the 'relevant
others' who Finch considered involved in displaying family needs to be
widened in multi-purpose settings as other authors in this volume have
also illustrated (McIntosh et al., Chapter 10).

The data used in my study came from a range of sources. A small-
scale empirical study was carried out in 2001 in which fieldwork was
split between two U.K. east coast seaside resorts; one in the south
and one in the north of England. In-depth interviews were carried
out with two samples, the first being people who were currently running hotels, pubs and boarding houses and were bringing up or had
recently brought up their families in such establishments. These
interviews were carried out with at least one proprietor and (where
there was more than one) both where this was convenient and appropriate. In addition, when children living in the establishments were
available and willing, they were included in the interview. This
resulted in data from fifteen parents and four children across eleven
establishments (seven hotels, two pubs and two boarding houses). In
the second sample a further six interviews were undertaken of individuals and couples who had raised their families in such establishments, or grew up in them in the 1960s and 1970s (four hotels, one
pub and one boarding house). Access was negotiated first by letter
through local Hotelier Associations and later by snowballing. All the
interviews except two (on the interviewees' request) were taped and

transcribed. Finally, secondary data analysis was carried out on fifty oral-history interviews relating to participation in the tourist industry in one northern seaside town during the early and middle twentieth century.[1]

Displaying (business) families

The hospitality establishments included in my study were family-run hotels, not just family hotels (that is, for patrons to attend with their families) so the families of the proprietor(s) were living *in situ*. This created a setting where there was a family/business interface and where, as mentioned above, the audience for any display was complex and multiple, making the process more complex than that in solely domestic settings (cf. Seymour 2007).

The concept of 'displaying family' refers to a public presentation of family practices which is both for family members and for other social actors. As Finch says, the display defines family composition and family cohesion: 'These are my family relationships, and they work' (2007: 73). Yet the interviewees in my study were also displaying that 'this is my family business and it works'.

This multiplicity of activities has been discussed by Morgan (1996) in relation to family practices and he acknowledges that the same activity can be labelled in a variety of ways (for example, gendered, work, generational) depending upon the audience, which can include researchers. His discussion also confirms that interactive activities can have more than one intent. In the case of the family-run hospitality setting, this means addressing both business and family agendas. Family members will be carrying out activities which are part of everyday family life but which also signal that theirs is a family-run business. This leads to the potential display of several activities which could be conceived as a continuum from family practices, through family practices in a business setting, family-business practices to business practices.

Examples of these different forms of display can be seen in the accounts of my interviewees from those where all actions were seen as family practices:

> [Of daughter's actions] Well, it's part of family life, she's part of the family so she does it. (Interview 14, female boarding-house owner)

Through carrying out family practices in a business setting:

> ... it was just the right sort of hotel ... 'cos the seaside hotel brings all that sort of family trade. As if you were say, in London, in a business hotel, that would be a totally different kettle of fish ... nor would customers want to mix with children would they? Discuss business, they don't want a snotty nosed child with a toffee apple. (Interview 7, female boarding-house owner)

To displays of family-business practice which allowed the emphasis to be on the family-run element of the establishment:

> The family I think helped towards the business in that the families staying in hotels, they sort of [know] you will run a family and so understand what their problems would be. (Interview 5, male ex-hotel owner)

In these cases, family members could also include household pets (Gabb 2008; Gabb this volume), because they also contribute to constructions of homeliness and intimacy in the hospitality establishment:

> The little dog wants to come in [to the guest areas]. I let her in and everything stops...*[A] touch of home* ... Rather than us being these figures kind of behind the business, I think it makes us more real to them, you know, *we are a family*. (Interview 17, female hotel owner, my emphasis)

The final point on the continuum is business practices and for some interviewees there was complete separation of the two arenas, spatially and cognitively:

> We always kept it separate. We had to come in through the pub 'cos we didn't have a separate entrance. That was something that we always tried to keep, you know straight through and up, so the kids didn't get to hang around inside the pub. (Interview 9, male ex-publican)

Within the international research literature on commercial homes, this potential continuum is recognised, often (as Hall does in his work on New Zealand) using the concept of the servicescape (Bitner 1992; Hall 2009). The family become elements of the servicescape (the shared physical setting of a business) or, as Carmichael and McClinchey (2009) suggest in their study of rural areas, the commercial home (and its occupants) present a continuum from homescape to servicescape (also Lynch et al. 2009c: 206).

To complicate matters further, individual family members could be simultaneously displaying different practices through the same activity. For example, children may be less conscious of the need for display of family-business practices and simply be carrying out displays of family practices in a business setting as that is their home. This may be age-related and it has been proposed that the stage in the family life cycle or family events will be significant factors determining the nature of the guests' stay (Lynch et al. 2009b: 5). Yet several authors in this volume (Almack, Short and Doucet) emphasise that degrees of intensity relating to the need to display families may be less influenced by stages in the life cycle than by resistance to normative ideals.

It can be argued that, in the single-location home/workplace, the dimensions of display which have been discussed as occurring in the purely domestic setting are heightened. The forms of display in a family-run business are not necessarily different, but they become *essential* rather than optional due to the commercial nature of the context. In addition, they must be made absolutely explicit to ensure that they are 'effective'; that is, that the audience appropriately constitute (read) the meanings they are intended to convey (Finch 2007: 66). Displaying family therefore becomes a complex and, apparently, paradoxical mix of presentation and reticence – the family has to be highly visible but not publicly privileged over guests. Thus, family members must be hyper visible while also, on certain occasions, exhibiting 'displayed reticence'. In addition, 'the family' in a family-run establishment is part of the business discourse, hence this again suggests that displays are mandatory and that degrees of intensity are not just about the current family form or stage in the life cycle, but also the context in which they are taking place; in this instance, the business establishment. Hence, the resonance of my findings with other authors' statements in this volume (particularly Doucet, but also Almack and Short) that intensity is not necessarily about events in the lives of individual families, but can be about being perceived by others as going against normative ideals. Here that would constitute not living out family life in a purely domestic setting. In addition, families in commercial homes have cyclical changing identities rather than necessarily longitudinal ones. These are diurnal, weekly, and seasonal and may include the transition from a long-term family member to a hospitality worker. For each transition, change must be actively demonstrated and renegotiated as Finch (2007: 72) suggests but in an iterative rather than linear manner. In the section following I show how the families in my study used inventive and varied ways to display their multiple roles and paradoxical positions.

Essential family displays for pubs and commercial homes

It is first worth reiterating, as Finch says, that all relationships require an element of display to sustain them as family relationships (2007: 71). Thus, the guest families on holiday in commercial homes will be displaying to other family members and also, in public places such as lounges and dining rooms, to a wider audience. Similarly, the families in my study will be displaying their families as well as displaying their family-business, but it is this latter activity that requires the curious combination of hyper visibility (to emphasise the family nature of the business) with displayed reticence (to show that the guests always come first).

Displaying hyper visibility

One interviewee who had grown up in a pub remembered:

> As people come in, you know my mum ... the landlady welcoming them in type of thing.

But he also noted that the family would provide moral support if there was violence in the pub:

> I can't remember how the word went round but we ended up hearing there was something going on, I don't know if we were upstairs at the time and we came downstairs to watch them behind the bar. (Interview 1, adult son of ex-publican)

In hospitality establishments family health matters which may normally occur in private became a public issue:

If they had measles everybody had to know about it, age three or four. (Interview 7, female ex-hotel owner)

Although, in contrast, the oral-history data from the early-to-mid twentieth century cited an example of a family whose children developed chicken pox and were removed from a boarding house to their grandparents' loft so as not to lose the booking and hence valuable income.

Mealtimes are often seen as the sine qua non of family activities (James 2007; Southerton 2009). Per Finch all families display in public restaurants, but this is especially so for the host family as they form part of the servicescape (Carmichael and McClinchey 2009; Hall 2009; Lynch et al. 2009c). At mealtimes the families in the study were opening up their behaviour to public scrutiny (Carmichael and McClinchey 2009: 75) showing they were capable of acting like a family in a public setting in a way which provided reinforcement even if no one external to the group gave specific feedback. They were 'doing family' but they were doing family as the proprietor family in a business environment and relevant others were supporting the social meanings thereby established. Hence as one ex-hotelier describes:

For many years we had a table in the dining room with the guests. That began to fail after maybe a year or two, because, you know, you've got no privacy, your children wanted to have a tantrum, they'd have to do it in public. (Interview 7, female ex-hotel owner)

The hyper visibility of displaying family-business practices also includes acting as role models to other families in the dining room in both attire and behaviour. As Hall notes in his New Zealand study, family members in the servicescape are used to demonstrate to guests how to behave 'properly' (2009: 69), while other authors discuss the censure in the United Kingdom on wearing pyjamas in public rooms (Benmore 2009: 122). The communication of desired standards, while attempting to be hospitable, constitutes a complex transactional relationship. Heaphy (Chapter 2) discusses how display can be used to demonstrate respectability, normative class and desired manners. It attempts to set the 'tone' for the hotel; for example, whether or not diners can wear curlers or shorts in the dining room. Within the tourism and hospitality literature such behaviours are considered to be performances (Darke and Gurney 2000; Di Domenico and Lynch 2007: 118–9; Lynch et al. 2009a). Finch, however, wishes to distinguish between performativity, performance and display, considering the former to be about individual identity whereas performance is about face-to-face interaction in which the performer remains an actor. She argues that display differs in that it conflates the actor and the audience (and there may not be feedback). It does have to be questioned as to whether very young children are actively displaying, however it is entirely possible that they are being 'displayed'. The concept of display allows a consideration of the uncritical acceptance of performance in the tourism and hospitality literature and suggests it can add a useful development to research in these disciplines.

Displayed reticence – visible as family member, not as guest

The phrase used in the title to this chapter 'Family Hold Back' (or, perhaps more cryptically to the uninitiated, 'FHB') is one used by (usually) parents to signal to family members that guests should have first choice and as many servings as they wish at mealtimes. It conveys the idea that, if there is any shortage of resources, it is family members who should bear these rather than those invited into the home. As such, it may seem at odds with the idea that parents would seek the best for their children but it does fit in with ideas of offering hospitality, particularly those of 'altruistic giving' (Selwyn 2000: 21). Unlike in private homes, where 'FHB' may be a muttered injunction which could embarrass the hosts with its implication of insufficient provisions, in commercial homes it could be argued that family reticence is a necessary requirement and one which needs to be explicitly demonstrated and read effectively as such by the guests. Hence the business family will need to be involved in 'displayed reticence' to counterpoint their hyper visibility as family members. It must be made clear to the audience of guests (and staff) that, although present, family members are in no way privileged over paying customers. This displayed reticence is different from the absences of display discussed in Almack's and Hughes and Valentine's chapters in this volume, as it is a specialised form of display rather than a lack of it.

Interviewees spoke of numerous occasions and events when they were publically present in the establishment but not involved in the guests' activities:

> [I remember] Watching entertainment, not joining in. (Interview 4, adult son of ex-hotel owner)

> Behind the bar, you know, at night time, went down for a bag of peanuts or half a lager and lime or whatever and used to stand behind the bar a lot as well and watch the pub and listen to music. (Interview 1, adult son of ex-publican)

> She sat there quite contentedly really all afternoon, watching everybody else. (Interview 7, female ex-hotel owner)

Mealtimes feature again in the accounts as a public site of displaying family and one where displayed reticence could be made transparent. This included being seated at the 'worst' table (near the kitchen or toilets), being served last or not having the choicest foods.

> Poor souls. They used to get plonked on table while we were serving meals and I just saying to somebody this morning in hindsight we should have fed them first and then we wouldn't have had them saying 'I'm hungry, Mummy, I want something to eat' and my Dad'd be saying 'Oh for goodness sake, shut up till we're finished serving the visitors', you know.

> ... They were sat at the table waiting as soon as we got the pudding out then we served them with their dinner and they could get on with theirs 'cos we had a great big serving table so they used to sit at the back of the serving table. You just had to fit it in and work around things. (Interview 12, female hotel owner)

> Family meals, *after the guests always*. Mum and Dad had theirs in the dining room with the guests. (Interview 5, male ex-hotel owner)

Children of hoteliers were aware of these priorities (and that they differed from 'normal' families) but recognised them as an essential component of growing up in a family hotel.

I suppose sometimes I felt that the best things, whatever they were, the best cuts of meat for example, would go to the guests and, talking to other children, their parents would always try and get the best for the family. It's such a small quantity in terms of the whole, we managed without. (Interview 4, adult son of ex-hotel owner)

And not all parents or guests expected displayed reticence from these children:

[Of games night with guests] Did you ever have to not let them win?
Interviewee: No I didn't do that, I never did that no. I let them win and often the visitor would give them things as well, they'd give things that were their prizes that they'd won. (Interview 10, female hotel owner)
We did say to guests that were coming at Christmas that if the kids were humping sacks around at five in the morning, you know, they would be allowed to. I don't think they've ever been pushed out because of guests. (Interview 15, female boarding-house owner)

However, it could be argued that sometimes the priorities given to guests were more to do with their adult status than guest status. The quotations below could be interpreted as illustrating dimensions of power relating to age rather than to commerce or to a combination of both.

[The] TV [was] in [the] lounge and if they [daughters] were watching television the visitor would come in and just turn the programme over. They never thought the child was watching the television and they never thought to say 'Are you watching this?' (Interview 10, female hotel owner)

We did use the visitors' lounge but we had people who used to complain about us using *their* lounge. They didn't complain about the children using the lounge they just used to turn the station over on the telly. (Interview 10, male hotel owner)

If [child's] friends sit on [the] furniture out front [there's] no room for guests. (Interview 16, female hotel owner)

> If I'm talking to a guest he can't come and interrupt and if I'm talking to him a guest can interrupt. He's had to learn, you know, that the work has to come first. (Interview 6, female hotel owner)

> Whenever I came home the guest were always more important than me.

> ... but whether parental time and attention goes elsewhere, and I would think it could cause resentment to the children as it did to me. (Interview 13, adult son of ex-hotel owners and hotel owner)

In writing about the home as a place of consumption, Gurney (1999: 48) discusses 'power and resistance relations between household members and their guests'. His account does not include *paying* guests but it can be seen that the complex and socially sensitive relations which occur in private households when shared with non-family members can be magnified in commercial hospitality settings and hence require significant displays on the part of the business family.

Replacing display with invisibility

Some owners of family-run hotels, pubs and boarding houses chose not to make their family members, particularly children, hyper visible but did make them explicitly reticent. Others simply kept family life separate from their commercial activities, either by spatially separating the two areas, or by closing the business when there were family events. In these situations family members would be invisible rather than displaying reticence but this still led to some spatial and temporal constraints, for example:

> Couldn't use the bathroom just when you wanted to. You had to fit in and have it when guests were having their meal. (Interview 5, male ex-hotel owner)

Here, although not a display, interviewees were describing the multi-purpose activity of a family practice in a business setting.

Displaying families – always positive?

Morgan (1996: 192) reminds us that to recognise family practices as significant 'is not the same as saying that they are always positively evaluated'. Some of the experiences outlined previously, relating to displaying family in a single-location home/workplace, reinforce this statement. Yet, in her seminal article, Finch states that 'thus there is a real sense in which defining "my family" is also an evaluative statement about the positive character of these relationships' (: 70) while later outlining that the core message of displaying is 'these are my family relationships and they work' (2007: 73). The data presented in this chapter should go some way towards problematising this (overly?) positive presentation of displaying family. Although interviewees recognised some positive dimensions to the hyper visibility of being part of a family-run hotel/boarding house or pub, such as being spoiled for the former, or community recognition for the latter, they could provide many examples of more negative aspects, as in the following quotation:

> You'll say to your kids 'Get in there or you're getting a good hiding' and they [guests] say 'Oh you can't do that' and ... you're thinking 'Just keep out, it's my family'. (Interview 16, family member and hotel worker)

Although some guests had commented that hearing the host family arguing or the children being disciplined made the hospitality establishment even more like a 'real' family home, it was clear that most such actions were 'shushed up'. The danger with hyper visibility, especially with children, is that displaying family can reveal a family that doesn't work (by whatever normative standards of legitimacy are being utilised) and although 'the family' is recognised by the audience, the feedback is negative. In addition, parents sometimes considered that their children were more exposed to issues of sex and sexuality because they were growing up in single-location home/workplaces rather than in private homes and, as found by Di Domenico and Fleming (2009), had concerns about their ability to police such activities in what was their own household.

Conclusion

Looking at the empirical example of family-run hotels, pubs and boarding houses allows the application and testing of the concept of displaying family but also highlights areas where it can be interrogated and further developed. Many chapters in this volume, including Hughes and Valentine, show displaying family can be done just with family members, but this chapter suggests that it is particularly adaptable to situations where there are public, and potentially multiple, audiences.

In relation to the substantive topic of the commercial home or pub (and indeed other business settings), the ideas of hyper visibility and displaying reticence have proved useful dimensions of the concept and also allow the consideration of circumstances when display is not used, such as deliberate invisibility. The concept of displaying family allows researchers to differentiate between family practices in a business setting and family-business practices. In the case of the former, displaying family may not necessarily occur but the data suggest that, in the case of the latter, such displays are essential and must be unambiguous to prevent unfortunate commercial consequences. The application of the data to existing studies of commercial homes has shown the international applicability of the concept. While investigation of the tourism and hospitality literature has been shown to enhance the consideration of research on social relations and interactions, it also appears that the application of the concept of displaying family to this literature can develop and expand investigations of ways of 'producing social relations' in tourism and hospitality studies (Haldrup and Larson 2003: 24). As such, examination of this concept could contribute to an increased and productive cross-fertilisation of investigation between social sciences and tourism and hospitality research.

In consideration of the concept itself, it has been shown that in some settings participants are not only moving between 'doing family' and 'displaying family', but may be carrying it out in sites where it can be read as having multiple meanings depending upon the relevant others who make up the audience, or where multiple activities are being undertaken. As such, the examination of displaying family in such settings can contribute to the widening consideration of family practices in non-domestic settings (Seymour, forthcoming).

To interrogate the concept further, there needs to be more consideration of the potentially negative aspects of displaying family. What do participants mean when they try to convey that their family relationships work? How can this be unpacked to consider issues of quality, practicality and effectiveness? Researchers need to investigate further such negative aspects so that, as has happened with family practices, studies can attempt to capture the full spectrum of family life and intimate relationships, and show how the reality and ideology of both can be difficult to reconcile in everyday life.

Finally, this may be the point for sociologists beyond those of the family to assess the concept of display. This chapter has shown that what is being done in certain circumstances may be more than just a family display. Displays could be read as gendered, commercial, generational or they could, by quizzing different audiences, be used to reveal age-specific ways of reading the same activity. So there needs to be an investigation of how displaying family maps onto other practices and substantive areas of research. In this volume, Heaphy has proposed that displaying should be considered as applying, not just to families, but also to other intimate relationships. This chapter suggests we should go further and consider, not only its applicability to intimate relationships, but also to areas where family studies cross-cut other research interests and where other topics stand separate from those of the family.

Note

1. The interviews were funded by the Millennium Commission and conducted as part of the 'Looking Back, Looking Forward' project carried out by the North Yorkshire Museums Department. I am grateful to the project's organiser Karen Snowden, the interviewers and particularly the interviewees, who allowed their thoughts and words to be passed on to other researchers.

10

'I Know we Can't be a Family, but as Close as You Can Get'*: Displaying Families within an Institutional Context

Ian McIntosh, Nika Dorrer, Samantha Punch and Ruth Emond

Despite often expressed concerns over its apparent demise, the idea (or ideal) of 'the family' continues to exert a powerful presence within a range of contexts (McKie et al. 2005). As Weeks puts it:

> Family is a powerful and pervasive word in our culture, embracing a variety of social, cultural, economic and symbolic meanings; but traditionally it is seen as the very foundation of society. It is also a deeply ambiguous and contested term in the contemporary world, the subject of continual polemics, anxiety, and political concern about the 'crisis of the family'. (Weeks et al. 2001: 9)

We of course need to be wary about referring to 'the family' in the singular; Gittins (1993) suggests using the plural term 'families' in order to reflect its variety. Whilst this usefully acknowledges diversity, it is also important to consider what is meant by this dynamic and complex term 'family'. Despite recent critiques of the conventional family, there are still collective views of what families should look like that continue to dominate in many ways today:

> An *ideology* provides collective definitions of what a 'normal' family is thought to be, what is a 'proper' marriage, and what it means to be a 'good mother' or a 'good father'. Family ideologies are held out as ideal ways of living. (Cheal 2002: 72)

Ideas about the 'ideal family' are not unfamiliar to most people, as Gittens reminds us: 'It manifests just enough similarity to people's life situations to make it seem tangible and real to most' (1993: 165). Precise definitions of the family are, of course, notoriously difficult to come across but, even if often elusive, constructions of the family can be no less powerful and compelling. As VanEvery (1999: 178) highlights, '"family" also connotes ties of love and affection, commitment, and obligations whether these are formally recognised or not'. Thus, the power and presence of the family can be shown even within contexts and spaces which are, on the surface, not obviously amenable to attempts at creating family or family-like relations. This is the case within residential care homes for children and young people and is the focus of this chapter.

Families are recognised not just for what they are but what they do, such as sharing resources, caring, meeting responsibilities and fulfilling obligations (Silva and Smart 1999). Morgan (1996) argues that families are an on-going consequence of daily interactions, routines and transactions which may be both enabling and constraining. Given that it is recognised that there are diverse ways of 'doing family', Finch (2007) has introduced the concept of 'display' as a way of understanding the diversity and fluidity of contemporary family relationships. She emphasises that 'displaying' family is as important as 'doing' family. There is a need to 'display' family in order to demonstrate to others that one's actions and interactions are family practices which are recognised as such by others. This can be more important where relationships take a non-conventional form. Hence, the concept of display coincides with perceiving families as a qualitative relationship 'rather than a thing' (Morgan 1996: 186).

The typical setting for the family is, of course, the home, as expressed most obviously in the couplet family-home. Indeed the connection between the two terms is so commonplace that they are often used synonymously. More specifically, the private and domesticated space called 'home' is often defined in contradistinction to 'work'. The workplace is in many ways the antithesis of the family-home and the two spaces are often seen to be incommensurable. However, as Seymour (2007) notes in her discussion of the 'single location home/workplace', the two worlds and spaces of home and work can collide and this can pose problems for any attempts at maintaining and displaying 'family-like' relations and activities which are recognisable to actors as such. This is relevant for our discussion given that the residential home is clearly a workplace for staff and at the same time they are charged with making it a home for children. In addition, given the highly regulated and surveilled nature of many of the spaces within the residential care home, it is often viewed and experienced by staff and children as being an 'institution' in its operation and ethos (Dorrer et al. 2010).

These three often conflicting aspects of the residential care home – a workplace for staff, a 'home' for children and an 'institution' for both – can make attempts at creating interactions and experiences which are 'family-like' problematic. Despite this, such attempts are regularly made and can perhaps shed further light on the power of 'the family' as an ideal form of social relations and the ways in which it is used and evoked. As Gillis (1996) has proposed, while the contemporary families we live with have taken on a more fragmented and diverse nature, the imagined families we 'live by' have become powerful reference points. Indeed, the notion of the family operated as an exemplar of certain types of relations and had a heavy presence in the culture and daily routines across the three residential homes we studied. Constructions and representations of the family could have the effect of being a regular, if often vague and difficult to pin down, default ideal toward which there was a continuous gravitation. A key way in which the enactment of family ideals and values was attempted was via food and food practices, particularly those associated with mealtimes. As Jackson (2009: 1) notes; 'what we eat, how, when and where... provides a powerful way of observing changes in family life'. In this chapter we examine some of the ways in which food and food practices were central to efforts to create, and regularly display, 'family' relations and experiences and a 'home' or a 'homely' ambiance within the units.[1]

The study

Whilst the approaches and operational regimes of residential establishments in Scotland vary (see Table 10.1), their central function is to provide twenty-four–hour care and support to children who are unable to live within a family-home. The majority of these children will have been assessed by social work as 'at risk' of physical or emotional harm and/or who pose a potential risk to themselves or others. There may be some who are accommodated on a 'voluntary' basis; however, this too would in all likelihood require social work assessment. There are also residential units which provide twenty-four–hour

Table 10.1 The research settings

Characteristics	Wellton	Highton	Lifton
Age of children	9–13 years	12–16 years	14–18 years
Ethos	Focus on providing safety and structure; consistent implementation of clear boundaries and routines. Emphasis on children experiencing 'normal' family-like living and learning practical skills.	Focus on overcoming institutional characteristics, creating a relaxed environment, recognising diversity, offering choices. Emphasis on maintaining safety and developing independent living skills.	Focus on being 'family-like', creating connectedness, and building relationships. Emphasis on creating a sense of belonging rather than developing children's independent living skills.
Food Routines Shared mealtimes around the table	Tea (children make their own lunch supervised by adults)	Lunch and tea	Lunch and tea
Breakfast (some variation at weekend)	Prepared at staggered intervals to avoid clashes and delays	May be in their bedrooms or may take something to eat on way to school	Individualised routines between particular children and staff
Supper	Supper kept to a minimum; usually just juice in children's bedrooms as a means to settle them for the night.	Toast and cheese in the dining or living room. Prepared by children or staff.	Tea and toast in the living room. Other snacks if requested. Prepared by staff.

Participation			
Organisation of meals	Cook prepares tea on week-days. Care workers prepare meals when the cook is off.	Cook prepares lunch and tea at weekends and some weekdays. Assistant managers, domestic and care workers prepare meals when cook is off.	Cook prepares lunch and tea on week-days. Assistant managers, domestic and care workers prepare meals when the cook is off.
Who participates in the main meal	Care workers and children.	Care workers, cook, assistant managers and children.	Care staff, cook, managers, domestic and admin staff, and children.
Cleaning tasks	Cleaning rota: each child takes turns doing the dishes. Care workers contribute to cleaning.	Children expected to clean their own dishes. Care workers contribute to cleaning.	No expectations that children clean their own or others' dishes. Cook and domestic staff mainly responsible for cleaning.

care to children who require it as a result of physical or learning disability; this type of provision was not included in our study.

Data were generated using ethnographic techniques and involved three, twelve-week blocks of semi-participant observation in three residential children's homes (between three and six day-long visits per week, and some overnights). The data consisted of thirty-six weeks of field notes, overt audio recordings of mealtime interactions, forty-eight unstructured or spontaneously recorded interviews, forty-nine semi-structured interviews and twelve focus groups with children and staff from the three homes. In total sixteen children aged nine to eighteen (eleven boys and five girls) and forty-six members of staff (twenty-six women and twenty men including managerial staff, care workers, cooks, administration and domestic staff) took part in individual interviews and/or a focus group. The identities of the children's homes and our participants are protected by using pseudonyms and presenting only pen pictures of the homes ('Lifton', 'Wellton' and 'Highton') in Table 10.1. The research was guided by the British Sociological Association's Statement of Ethical Practice and was informed by established codes of ethics for researching with children (Alderson and Morrow 2004) and the previous work of Emond (2005) and Punch (2002). Data were analysed thematically facilitated by the computer package NVivo.

Displaying family

In her influential article, Finch defines family display in the following way:

> The process by which individuals, and groups of individuals, convey to each other and to relevant others that certain of their actions do constitute 'doing family things' and thereby confirm that these relationships are 'family' relationships. (2007: 73)

Finch sees such forms of display as being crucial for the 'nurturing and development of relationships' and for ensuring that '"family-like" qualities are positively established' (2007: 80). It has been suggested that the concept of 'displaying family' can be a useful 'orienting device to examine what might be going on below the surface of family lives' (Almack 2008: 1195). In her analysis of how

lesbian parent couples were seeking to gain recognition and validation of their family status, Almack (2008) illustrates how 'display
work' in the form of kinship-related activities arises, particularly in
contexts where the quality of family relationships can be subjected
to doubt or where there is a deviation from conventional understandings of what a family looks like. Such an intensified need to
engage in interactions and activities which have a family quality can
also prevail in residential children's homes. While staff in the three
homes in this study emphasised that they had no intention of trying
to replace the children's biological families, the majority also felt the
children had a right to experience childhood in an environment
that was as close to family as possible. Explanations of what good
residential care would consist of frequently entailed references to
practices of 'normal' families or the staff's own experiences of family
life. However, as we outlined previously, the public, institutional and
workplace nature of the settings in which care was provided could
also lead to a great deal of uncertainty about how relationships in
residential homes could be family-like. The residential care context
thus constitutes a challenge to taken-for-granted understandings of
what it means to be a family, a parent and a child.

Food practices offered socially recognisable rituals and routines
that could help make family-like qualities within the residential
home more identifiable and tangible. Conspicuous displays, such as
having a meal together around the table, could be experienced as
greatly rewarding by staff and children. When displays of such practices were unsuccessful, however, they could be seen as the markers
of a 'bad shift'. Below the surface of displays of doing family there
were thus often profound feelings of ambiguity.

What the brief descriptions of the ethos of each home in this study
(see Table 10.1) illustrate is that the level of commitment to being like
a family and consciously doing family-like things varied across the
three residential homes. However, what was always notable was the
continued significance and allure of constructions of the family and
this was evidenced in a general acceptance by many of the staff of
the therapeutic benefits of the creation of family-like relations. The
following comments illustrate this:

> I'd love it to be like a family. And I try my best to make it like a
> family home...I think you show that you actually care, and you

genuinely care. Make no mistake about it, I'm not here for the wages 'cause I could get better paid jobs out there. I want to be here and I want to try and make a difference to them. ...I try my best to make it as homely as possible, as much like a normal home. (Gail, care worker, interview, Highton)

What you're trying to do is run it almost like family home where you've got a routine, and the mealtimes come into this. (Geoff, care worker, interview, Lifton)

Children, too, spoke of positive experiences of being cared for by residential staff in terms of being like a family:

I just feel like they're more like a mum and dad, well like a family, to me than my mum and dad will ever be. [...] All the staff are caring and willing to help you, but if you like muck stuff up in Lifton they'll be like, they'll give you the chance to help. (Adam, young person, interview, Lifton)

Others explained to us that living in residential care is less than ideal, for example, by highlighting that mealtime practices lacked the familiarity of family meals. As Malcolm said:

Aye, I know Scott's cooking's nice, but once you've been in your own family home for quite a bit and you're used to a family home, and you're used to your family's cooking, when you get brought away from that it's just like basically sitting eating at your mate's house and that's fucking rancid. (Malcolm, young person, interview, Highton)

It was often taken as a given by many staff that the creation of a family-like atmosphere was positive and had therapeutic benefits. The strong moral force and presence of the family and family-home as an unquestionably 'good thing' resonated strongly with many of the staff in the three homes. Clearly, whilst homogenised and monolithic understandings of the family are misplaced empirically (Morgan 1996), what continues to persist in people's sense making is a dominant social representation (Moscovici 2000) of family anchored in ideas of constancy, closeness and support. As Jackson notes:

[The] image of the nuclear family remains a powerful normative social ideal, underpinned by strong institutional forces and capable of exerting considerable moral force. The strength of the family as an ideal is shown in our research on homeless men who sought to (re)create family-like relations though networks of fictive kin and through attempts to foster a homely, familial atmosphere in hostels and similar institutional settings. (2009: 3)

Thus, ideas of the (typically, nuclear) family can inform the actions of actors even within an environment not obviously amenable to the creation of a family such as a residential care home.

Food practices and displaying family

Residential care – on a policy and inter-personal level – is surrounded by ambiguity and uncertainty (McPheat et al. 2007; Smith 2009). This, in line with Finch's (2007) concept of displaying family, could result in an intensified need to gain validation of the quality of people's relationships. Food practices are closely associated with socially shared representations of the family and thus offer means for 'doing family' (see also Punch et al. 2010). Moreover, food practices invite interaction and can thus function as an arena in which 'doing family' can also be displayed to an audience, in our case an audience made up of a combination of children and/or staff. As Finch (2007) has argued, the act of recognition through an audience is crucial for display work to be successful.

A key way in which doing family was attempted across all of the residential homes was through regular and patterned mealtime routines. This could provide a form of 'normality' in the everyday experiences of the children:

There is structure and routine to the day that I think, em, resembles family time ... in a normal household. There's a getting up time, there's a breakfast time, there's a lunchtime, there's a dinner time, there's a going out in the evening and having your social time, there's a pick up time and there's a bedtime. (Linett, care worker, interview, Lifton)

The symbolically loaded act of sitting around the table together for a meal was a key and regular event. Yet it could be argued that such a practice is less typical in the average family house where meals often take place in the kitchen or in front of the television. Nevertheless, commensality, the practice of sharing food and eating together in a social group, has been recently described as 'central to defining and sustaining the family as a social unit' (Ochs and Shohet 2006: 37). As Victor highlights, this could be a new experience for many children entering residential care:

> I think it's just unwritten rules ... ask for things politely, you know, 'can you pass the salt please' and ... just the social niceties that go along with mealtimes. I mean I suppose a lot of our kids probably didn't have a structured family meal, so it's a bit of an alien experience. (Victor, care worker, interview, Lifton)

The role played by food and food practices within the inner life of the residential unit can be overlooked; for example, in Smith's (2009) otherwise comprehensive discussion of residential child care, food is not mentioned. However, in our research it was clear that mealtimes, accurately described by Fiese and colleagues as 'densely packed events' (2006: 87), were crucial in any attempts to create family experiences. As Larson and co-workers put it, 'For many families, mealtimes are the only time of the day when their members come together' and, further, that these 'shared meals have come to symbolize family unity' (2006: 1). Commensality, for some staff and children, is thus a 'normal' and an unstated 'expectation'. A member of staff put it succinctly: 'It's a ... family value that I've probably been brought up to do.' (Rob, care worker, interview, Wellton)

Similar comments, as the ones below, regularly emerged from all three of the residential care homes:

> I think mealtime is everybody sitting down and just sharing what they've done with their days, and just general catching up, just chatting [...] everybody's sitting down relaxing. [...] It feels like you're one big, happy family. And sometimes you can actually forget these kids aren't ... where they're from. It's just that relaxed. And I think the kids love it as well. (Sally, care worker, focus group, Highton)

> I think it is an expectation, but I think it's a good way of getting them all together and, if you like, a meeting point at one time in

the day for everybody, like a normal family would. (Gail, care worker, interview, Highton)

The family environment is when we have the lunchtimes and teatime where we have the table set and everybody, and it's a, it's just everyone sat down together. (Angela, care worker, focus group, Lifton)

Mealtimes then were seen to be crucial for blurring distinctions between staff and children and the work/home boundary. This is illustrated in the following comment:

Yeah, I mean it's, it's the centre of the unit, it's the one point in time where every body has a gathering point at lunch and evening meal where we sit and talk about our day and what's gone on and we tell jokes and we laugh and we moan about this, that and the other, and it's, it's a point in the day where everybody sits and that's the cook, the cleaner, the manager, the kids, everybody sits. That's your time to sit round when you just feel, yeah, it's... it's like a good family-home should be, you know, the old Sunday lunch, and we do that twice a day, which is great. (Derek, care worker, focus group, Lifton staff)

Fiese and colleagues point out the potential mealtimes have for regularly conveying meaning in that they can 'illustrate family identities and the creation of a sense of group membership... [they] are replete with symbolism, ranging from the types of blessings said, foods served, and even how seats are arranged' (2006: 68). Such benefits of eating together were largely accepted by many staff and the collective (albeit not always voluntary), everyday and routine nature of mealtimes gave it a power over other forms of socialising in the units, even if this potential was not always realised. The practice of displaying family is different from doing family in that it rests on a dialogic process of affirmation. That means a particular activity is not only done but it is directed at others and a response is in turn sought from others. Depending on what the response is, the addressor can deduce the extent to which the audience has understood and affirms the intended meaning or significance. The extract below provides an example of how staff used children's responses to their offers of food as an indicator that the children not only understood that such offers characterised the 'unit' as a place where you can feel at home, but also that they accepted and benefited from their care efforts. As Gail explains, the fact that children were anticipating dinner 'at home' was read as an acceptance of the mealtime values staff wanted to convey, which indicated to the staff that they were doing something right:

> I try my best to make it as homely as possible, as much like a normal home. [...] And very few kids come in here in the afternoon and don't shout, "What's for the tea?" and that's what you get in a normal home outside, isn't it? That's what you want to hear 'cause that's telling me they actually want to be here for their tea - they're not coming in and wanting to run back out that door again, and we're doing something right. (Gail, care worker, interview, Highton)

Our data suggest that the benefits of eating together and the role of food as a catalyst for fostering relations were indeed also taken on by children at times:

> I think it's good, actually. That's the best part. Everybody getting together like at teatime or something and just talking about their day, it's a kinda homely and family sorta thing. 'Oh I was at school the day' and all that type o' thing. (Colin, young person, interview, Lifton)

> Food does make you feel at home 'cause like you are all sitting around the table like one big family [...] I think it's good when Alice (the cook) comes and sits with us because then she feels part o' the family too. (Melanie, young person, interview, Lifton)

The examples above may illustrate that the doing and displaying of family-like relationships through mealtime practices could successfully create a feeling of togetherness and belonging (Punch et al. 2009). Beyond using mealtime practices to display family to each other and to the children, staff also used mealtimes to display their care work to outside audiences, as these events were considered to capture best what their work was about and that their work was different from other public services. Visitors such as members of the children's families, prospective foster parents, workers from other agencies, external service managers or the neighbourhood police officers would most commonly be invited to join a meal around the table. Of course, and somewhat paradoxically, such practices also rendered the residential home dissimilar from the typical family-home.

A further example of conspicuous display work was the annual Christmas buffet celebrated in one of the residential homes in this study. For staff and children at Lifton, the Christmas buffet played an important part in how this residential home constructed a family identity. Invitations for the buffet are sent out not only to local authority social workers and managers (as is the practice in some other residential homes), but to the teachers, friends and family of children living at Lifton, as well as to ex-residents and their families. Key elements of the event were the joint decorating of the house, the preparation of special foods cooked by staff collectively, and the display of holiday pictures from the past five years. As the children also helped with the preparations and invited others to see where they live, this event accomplished the criteria of participation and commitment that Silva and Smart (1999) highlight as necessary for the doing of family. Through inviting an external audience to see and evaluate in this way, Lifton could achieve a sense of continuity and connectedness. Such practices also served as a strong indicator of the staff's willingness to care beyond the prescribed duties of their paid employment. In the residential care context, because it can be hard to measure or demonstrate the quality of care provided, visible and tangible displays of 'doing family', such as sitting around the table together for meals, can enable staff to reassure themselves and others that they are providing an acceptable level of care.

Displays of family could, however, also be unsuccessful or go wrong. Not all children attributed significance to eating around the table together, as this comment by Alex illustrates:

> I don't really enjoy it, seeing everybody. It doesn't bother me if I see anybody. (Alex, young person, interview, Highton)

Others felt strongly that mealtimes around the table could only be associated with 'being together' if your actual family and friends were present. Callum's view was that in order to enjoy mealtimes he should be allowed to invite his friends to participate.

Nika: How about in here? Do you think it's [food] bringing people together in here?
Callum: Nah.
Nika: But people are sitting together, does that not count?
Callum: Nuh.
Nika: Why not?
Callum: 'Cause it has to be family and stuff.
Nika: It has to be family?
Callum: And friends. (Callum, young person, interview, Wellton)

Staff in this residential home, however, felt that the often challenging dynamics of mealtimes should not be displayed to friends. At difficult times in the residential homes, children frequently resisted attending mealtimes at the table or subverted staff expectations in regard to table manners and behaviour during meals. In such ways children could demonstrate their understandings of their relationships with staff in terms of an oppositional, us-versus-them, position (see also Punch et al. 2009). Thus, despite recognising that sitting at the table together for mealtimes could be 'family-like', and that this may be the aim of staff, many of the children resisted the notion of the residential unit being their home and could co-opt the setting for their own purposes.

Family display and ambivalence

Although ideas of an 'average' family and a 'normal' home were routinely used as reference points across all the residential homes, there was a great deal of ambivalence evident amongst staff and children in relation to the creation of a family-like atmosphere in the units:

> ...this is not their home and I would never patronise them by making out that we are a substitute for their home. We're just here to serve a purpose, which is to help them, whether it's getting back to their parents eventually [...] we're not their family. (Liam, care worker, interview, Highton)

We can see from the above quote that despite the recognition that the creation of family relations is problematic it was clear that, even if it was largely absent, the family as an ideal is still being invoked and can become a datum point from which relations in the unit are assessed and measured.

Many of the staff, though, were very conscious that the ability to indulge in meaningful displays of family tended to be limited and compromised by having to operate within what was recognised as the institutional confines of a residential home. Smith uses the notion of the 'milieu' to explore the often hard to define but powerful ethos of a residential care home:

> This overall medium created when staff and resident groups come together in a particular physical environment is referred to as the milieu. The concept is not particularly tangible ... it is the 'feel' of a place ... while it might be hard to measure [it] is likely to have a profound effect on those who live and work there. (Smith 2009: 87–8)

From our research the idea/notion of an 'institution' was regularly invoked to describe and explain the ambience and routines of the residential units. The following comments are illustrative of this:

> It's an institution. Now, we can make it as comfortable and as reasonable as we can, and to minimise all these kind of impacts, but to kid on that it's their home, that's an insult. (Scott, cook, interview, Highton)

> It's not ideal, pretending to be a home but you can't get away from the fact that we are an institution, there's no getting away from it. (Iain, care worker, interview, Highton)

> We can't make it completely average or ordinary because we need to have boundaries and structures and just by the very nature of having those it becomes institutionalised, it becomes, eh, regimented and routines that you wouldn't expect to find in an everyday family situation. (Vinnie, care worker, interview, Wellton)

The children were also aware of the ways in which life in the residential units did not always measure up to their understandings of family and home life:

> *Nika:* Do you think children think of Wellton as their home?
> *Natalie:* No. We got our own home. This is not where we belong. We got somewhere else. I am only here because my mum can't look after me.

Nika: So how do you think of here then?

Ross: I don't like it (Natalie and Ross, young persons, joint interview, Wellton)

A consequence of this institutional 'milieu' is that initiating and maintaining family display are likely to be more structured than Finch's (2007) and Morgan's (1996) analysis might allow, as they tend to emphasise the fluid nature of relations when displaying family. In the residential care setting, generally there involved much more of an imposition of constructions of family, albeit one that can be resisted and played out by children to some extent as the previous quotes indicate. As Silva and Smart point out:

> The focus on the ideas of 'doing' family as opposed to 'being' in a family demands participation and renewed commitment from individuals. (1999: 8)

The commitment to doing and displaying family varied across the units and over time. For example, some attempts to create family-like relations at mealtimes would falter or breakdown completely as a consequence of the tension and anxieties that develop through eating together around a table:

> From the young people's point of view not all of them want to eat in front of each other...They don't like that sort of community thing (laughs) they...they just want to be alone and have their meal. And that's, you know, that's fair enough. I think generally that sort of family orientated thing around the table is a good thing in a lot of ways. (Geoff, care worker, interview, Lifton)

> It's a kind of sense of identity, everyone, the staff and young people sit together and it's just...I don't know if I would go as far as to say it replicates the whole family situation...I don't think I've ever been in anyone's house when it's been mealtime and the kids have told the parents to, "Go fuck themselves," and "Fuck you", jump up on their feet and just...this barrage of abuse that the staff get. At the same time I think we're trying to show the importance of sitting together, saying this is what we do at mealtimes in our society, in our culture, and this is how you conduct yourself at the table, 'cause it will be part of their life up 'til they're seventeen

years old or whatnot. And just sit and have a conversation if we can. And sometimes as well topics can be raised in units, like the break-ins recently, the money being stolen, so you can address topics. (Liam, care worker, interview, Highton)

Sitting at the table, talking about the day's events, and playing out the roles prescribed in the act of doing family were all activities that were prone to breaking down. This is particularity the case within environments as complex as the residential care home. Indeed, mealtimes could be used as a forum for raising institutional concerns rather than partaking in family-like conversations. Spaces could also take on different meanings for residents and staff and they could have varying degrees of access and systems of boundary management. The kitchen, for example, was generally a clearly demarcated area which is highly regulated and managed and as such is the clearly 'institutionalised' space within the units. The bedrooms are often the most obviously domesticated private space. Communal living areas were marked with a degree of ambivalence and negotiation over their use. Similarly, eating areas could involve juxtaposing elements of strong surveillance on the one hand (McIntosh et al. 2010) and more relaxed attempts at family display on the other. Understandings of family were thus variously contested and accepted as people interacted through the different spaces and contexts in the home and, as we have seen, were often played out via food. A member of staff reflects on the subtleties involved:

I don't see a need for them to all be round the table like a tea time situation. Em, I think it's good for them to be able to go in and prepare something for themselves...and be able to manage that kind of thing, whereas other staff may just prepare something so that all the kids are sat round the table together again. So I would tend to manage it that it was more relaxed, and there's maybe one or two of them up at the breakfast bar, one or two of them at the table, one or two of them watching telly, that kind of way, depending on what's happening and what's going on. ... Creates less of this false big family kind of thing. (Claire, care worker, interview, Wellton)

An important way in which the residential home is experienced differently by staff and children is as a consequence of it being a workplace for staff, albeit an unusual workplace. The ideal of creating a 'home-like' environment – essentially, doing 'home' at work meant that, for staff, the work/home binary was rendered ambiguous and conflicting (see also Dorrer et al. 2010). By way of illustration a member of staff commented on the problem of having work breaks:

> They're not [breaks], you're still working, you're still with the kids. The only time you can go away on your own is if you smoke. (Rachel, care worker, interview, Highton)

Often only mealtimes without children present were considered a true break from work. In all three homes, food or beverages were used to structure time in terms of the alternation between professional, task-focused periods and relaxed, personal time. Some staff at Highton and Wellton described negative eating experiences as highlighting the difference of care homes from other workplaces:

> If you were in your own home you would eat when you wanted and have snacks when you wanted, so...you're the adult here, you're not one o' the kids and because you don't get breaks you do get that leeway to go and get a snack or whatever, even though you're still supervising and whatever, but the kids sometimes say, 'You're eating a yoghurt, how can I no get one?', but at the end of the day it's your job, you've got to keep yourself fuelled, if you know what I mean. (Cindy, care worker, interview, Wellton)

A central concern of staff was working within a framework of health and safety regulation. This was seen to be a major barrier to creating a non-institutional milieu and losing the connotations of a workplace environment:

> Ehh, well, I suppose you're more governed by health and safety things here, aren't you. You know, knives are locked away in cupboard and...and there's good reason for all of these things, you know...so I guess, kinda food, hygiene, health and safety, access to things at the time that you want it, you know. In my household if anybody wanted something to eat at three o'clock in the morning or come a-wandering through and just help themselves

to that. That can't happen in the same way here because that impacts on other young people. (Alana, care worker, interview, Lifton)

This reflects the tensions for staff between catering for individual children's needs and managing the safety and interests of the resident group. Thus, whilst many attempts to display family were made, especially by staff, it was recognised that in practice this could be very difficult to achieve, particularly given the tensions of a residential unit being simultaneously a place of work, home and institution.

Conclusion

The family practices approach as initiated by Morgan (1996) is a trenchant and influential critique of the more structural and fixed understandings of the family. However, the extent of the agency of individuals to create fluid family forms through everyday interaction can be exaggerated to some extent particularly when attempts to create family are made away from the normal setting for the family – the private home.

Within the residential homes' somewhat idealised forms of 'family-like' activities, relationships and behaviours were frequently adhered to by young people and staff, the motivation for this was often wholly positive attempts to build relationships and prepare children for life outside of the unit (Punch et al. 2009). The extent to which the children could accommodate or reject such attempts to imitate or engender a family ethos or family-like experiences also varied across the units and with each child. Staff also had an ambivalent relation to the creation of a family-home. There was of course no sense in which clearly structured family roles were mechanically imposed upon young people and staff, but neither was it the case that such roles and idealisations of the family were in every case resisted completely. As is the case within 'regular' family-homes, notions of the family were contested and negotiated across time and space and were regularly played out over food practices within the residential homes. Powerful representations (Jovchelovitch 2006; Moscovici 2000) and metaphors of 'the family', however, loomed large in the life of the units – particularly around mealtimes – and often took on the appearance of social facts that constrained and limited behaviour, if only to set agendas for subsequent resistance and denial.

The residential unit combines elements of a domestic space, a workplace and aspects of institutionalism. Within such a complex context the creation of a recognisable 'family' ambience and family-like experiences were rendered problematic on a daily basis. Given this, the extent to which family can be 'done' in a range of different contexts can thus be limited, particularly if agents are drawing upon dominant discourses of 'the family' as part of any display. As a member of one of the staff notes, they are, 'trying to bring a sort of family-type dynamic to it, that sometimes can be quite difficult in a residential setting' (Garry, care worker, interview, Wellton). What is remarkable is, given the above limits, how often attempts at family display are made and the key role that food and food practices play in striving to achieve this.

Notes

* Will, care worker, interview, Lifton.

1. We will refrain from using inverted commas around family and home, and related terms, from this point.

Part III
Afterword

11
Exploring the Concept of Display in Family Relationships

Janet Finch

In my initial exploration of the concept of 'displaying families' I posed the question: Does this concept add something valuable to the sociological tool kit (Finch 2007: 79)? I am therefore very pleased that other distinguished scholars have wanted to take up this question, in respect of families and personal relationships. The collection of articles in this volume offers a rich and stimulating range of reflections on the concept and its applications. It most certainly moves forward the sociological enterprise as well as our understanding of these most intimate contexts for social interaction.

In providing some brief reflections on the articles in this collection, I note that there are varying ways in which different authors have approached the topic of display, as well as a wide range of substantive examples and empirical data which have been deployed.

Applying the concept

Several authors in this volume have taken the concept of display and applied it to data from studies which were already in progress. These represent a variety of situations pertaining to families and personal relationships. Different types of settings for the development of relationships are explored; for example, ethnically mixed families (Haynes and Dermott); lesbian parents (Almack); residential settings (McIntosh et al.); and parenting especially fathering (Doucet). Different types of interaction and family dynamics are explored using the concept of display; for example, expression of emotional attachment (Gabb); the process of grandparents 'coming out' as having a grandchild with lesbian parents (Almack); and the re-working of relationships when one person in a family is trying to withdraw from problem gambling (Hughes and Valentine).

The application of the concept of display to these very varied situations serves to shed new light on them, according to each of the authors. It is notable that none of the studies referred to here was designed with the concept of display at its inception. So, what does the concept bring to the interpretation of data, and to analysis of the circumstances being explored?

One theme drawn out by these examples is that the concept of display aids understanding of *how relationships work over time*. Thus Almack considers the kinship context of lesbian parenting and the implications for grandparents in particular. For those who had not previously acknowledged publicly that their daughter was in a lesbian relationship, even though they may have been supportive, the birth of a child requires a reassessment. This event changes the circumstances in which families relate to each other and also how individuals present and explain their family relationships to others. Almack uses the concept of display to analyse the processes whereby grandparents reassess the ways in which they 'come out' as having a lesbian parent-couple within their kin network.

Hughes and Valentine also focus on changed circumstances within families, though of a different nature. Their study concerns individuals who are self-defined as problem gamblers, and who have decided that they are going to overcome the habit. This entails the re-working of identity, of intimate relationships and of living practices as others in the household and kin network support the former problem gambler and adjust their relationship to him or her. The authors describe this as a necessary process of partial infantilisation in order to overcome the habit, especially in the removal of all control over money, followed by a gradual return to normal adult responsibilities and rights. They use the concept of display to consider this process over time, in which there is an absolute requirement to find new ways of displaying the continuing meaningful nature of family relationships despite the infantilisation of one party. In due course, the process of 'earning' the right to return to adult status also entails displaying relationships as they undergo a further adjustment.

Each of these studies uses the concept of display, in the analysis of empirical data, in ways which serve to draw out a sociological insight, namely that it is important to deploy analytical tools which illuminate the consequences for relationships of the passage of time. Time also enters the analysis in a different way in two other studies in this volume, which focus on the significance of *moments in relationships,* and the importance of recognising those moments. Hayes and Dermott, drawing on their study of ethnically mixed families, make use of my discussion of degrees of intensity in the need for display, as does Doucet. I argued that changes in the circumstances of one or more individuals can trigger the need to re-specify and reconfirm family relationships. Thus, any family may experience times when there is a heightened intensity in the need to display family relationships (Finch 2007: 72).

Hayes and Dermott argue for the value of focusing on degrees of intensity in the need for display in understanding relationships within ethnically mixed families, because it highlights those moments when ideas about family are created and recreated. They use the example of wedding arrangements. Frequently the subject of extensive discussion in all families, in ethnically mixed families the planning of a wedding may require a much greater degree of reflection and renegotiation as widely differing national, religious or family traditions are brought together. In the process, at these moments in time, family relationships are refashioned.

Drawing on a different setting, Gabb's article also uses the concept of display to pinpoint the importance of 'moments' in time. Her study concerns the impact of sexuality on families (both lesbian and heterosexual) who have children. In her discussion of the difficulties of researching issues concerning the 'interior' of family life, she highlights the particular challenges, literally, of recognising men's demonstration of emotional attachment. Fathers commonly desire, she argues, to be both emotionally attached to their children and to be seen to be so attached, but a combination of factors limits their repertoire for displaying this. Thus 'for many men their emotions and their relational worlds can all too easily fail to register on cultural and analytical radars'. As a result researchers may not understand the meaning of what they are seeing and hearing, nor may others within the family network or external to it.

In these diverse ways the use of the concept of display – retrospectively, in studies where the data had already been collected – serves to remind us that it is important sociologically to understand family relationships as moving and changing over time. Pivotal moments in relationships only have significance because they are part of a process in which relationships have a past and an anticipated future, as well as a present.

Developing the concept

A number of the authors in this volume have taken up my invitation to develop the concept of display, analytically and conceptually, as well as to apply it. They have done so in various ways, often by linking the concept to others already commonly in use in the analysis of family relationships. Several authors, for example, draw out some additional points about gender and how gender relations map onto display, linking it, for example, to concepts such as emotional labour. This is certainly a dimension which would repay further work.

Using a different example, Heaphy considers the concept of display alongside the concept of scripting, drawing on a social interactionist tradition which sees intimate relationships not simply as 'following' scripts but also as creating them, with the script emerging and evolving through the interaction. He poses an interesting question about how examples of display, in the context of intimate relationships, are scripted. By linking these two concepts, he argues, we can ask illuminating questions about how relational displays draw on wider cultural meanings in the dynamic processes of social interaction. Personal scripts are linked with cultural scripts in a dynamic way, and thus 'new relationship stories' emerge.

In this discussion Heaphy is opening up important questions about how display actually happens in live social interactions. Do people make it all up as they go along? Are displays 'wholly creative', in his terms? Or, is displaying family relationships using cultural signals which are 'wholly given' – deploying gestures, words or symbols which are widely understood to denote empathy, contrition, affection and so on – within a given culture? In their article on displaying motherhood for first-time mothers, Kehily and Thomson also raise questions about how interpersonal displays are linked to wider cultural meanings, in this case with 'imagined families', those representations of family which abound in popular culture and serve to influence personal understanding and practices.

In concluding that relational display is a combination of the 'given' and the 'creative', Heaphy's analysis suggests some new lines of empirical enquiry, which could focus on how this combination actually operates for different individuals, and in different circumstances. Are there circumstances, for example, where there is more scope for display to be creative (in Heaphy's terms), or even where there is a requirement to be creative rather than to draw on 'given' elements?

Similarly the conceptual developments progressed in Hayes and Dermott's article also suggest new lines of empirical enquiry. They focus on developing the concept of audiences for displaying family, and argue that this illuminates questions about 'who matters' as an audience, in their case as an audience for displaying relationships that work well in ethnically mixed families.

They conclude that there is a multiplicity of potential audiences – parents, grandparents, friends, institutions such as schools – which are important in that they serve to shape the meaning of family practices. This leads them to argue that the concept of display needs to be developed to ensure that it does not over-emphasise individual agency and control over social interactions. This needs to be balanced with an understanding of how individual agency can be both shaped and constrained by the need to convey social meaning to a given audience. Indeed in some cases they see particular audiences (social workers or teachers, for example) as 'imposing' types of interaction – ways of behaving towards each other, for instance – on ethnically mixed families.

Whereas some of this analysis may move a little far beyond the concept of display, the significance of particular audiences, and the way in which they shape display, opens up further empirical questions about how display works in practice, and in different settings [see also Seymour and McIntosh et al., this volume].

Moving beyond the concept of displaying families in a different way, Heaphy poses a question about whether the concept of display potentially applies to other types of relationship, not simply within families.

That may well be an interesting line of enquiry. However, in the article which stimulated this volume, I grounded my theoretical case for the concept of display in Morgan's (1996) analysis of family practices where the emphasis shifts from 'being' a family to 'doing' family things. Families are understood, in this analysis, as sets of activities involving specific individuals, which take on social meaning associated with 'family'. Building on this analysis, I argued that families need to be 'displayed as well as done', focusing on the processes by which particular actions, words or gestures get connected with wider systems of social meaning (Finch 2007: 66–7). Thus my theoretical basis was grounded specifically in *family* relationships. Any extension of the concept of display to other types of relationships would require different theorising, albeit possibly with some common elements.

Critiquing the concept

Debate and dissent are the lifeblood of sociology, the means by which advances are made in those concepts and theoretical approaches which underpin our understanding of social life. My article on displaying families has generated debates and critiques of the concept, reflected in this collection.

Gabb questions the rather positive tone which is set in my discussion which, in her view, could be taken to imply that all examples of display are both recognisable and recognised and, in that sense, are successful in conveying social meanings. She cites examples which are both commonplace and important: a father building a wardrobe for his teenage daughter, a middle-class woman whose regular references to 'a cup of tea and a chat' were her shorthand way of describing how she sustained connections with various members of her family – her 'gift of intimacy'. The very commonplace nature of such actions may not easily be recognised as having significance for nurturing family relationships, Gabb argues. She makes a good point here. My article did not explore, to any depth, the possibility of 'unsuccessful' or misrecognised displays. This is an area which certainly would repay further development.

Questioning a slightly different aspect of my analysis, Heaphy argues that the concept of display is about 'claiming' family relationships, but that I have failed to recognise that some claims are more immediately validated than others. He argues that the concept requires a fuller understanding of diversity and difference in the context of relationships, how this relates to socio-cultural and political power, and the consequences for analysing display in family and other relationships. Invariably, he argues, 'it is those actors and relationships that most closely approximate to cultural ideals of 'normal' families whose displays are likely to be recognised, legitimated and validated' (Chapter 2).

Whilst I entirely accept the substantive point about diversity and legitimacy, I see that as a somewhat different issue from the areas which I was seeking to open up in the concept of display. Implicit in Heaphy's argument is the assumption that displaying family is equivalent to making claims for respectability or conventionality. This was not part of my argument. On the contrary, I set out the case for understanding family display in part by emphasising the fluid and diverse nature of contemporary families. I argued that, in many contemporary families, the contours of what constitutes 'my family' for any individual are not necessarily obvious or easy to identify, hence the need to demonstrate actively that certain relationships are important and meaningful – to show that 'This is my family and it works' (Finch 2007: 69–70). However, it is also possible that, in Heaphy's terms, such displays are not always 'legitimated and validated' as reflecting a cultural ideal of the normal family. We may need other concepts for analysing the latter process. The concept of display was explicitly intended to add to the sociological toolkit, not to replace all the other tools.

Displays and audiences

A common theme running through many of the articles in the collection, and in my discussion herein, relates to 'audiences' for display. I put this in quotation marks because the metaphor of the theatre is one which I find limiting to the analysis of displaying families, for reasons which I examine in my original article (Finch 2007: 76–7). However, the ways in which examples of display are *experienced, observed and understood by others* is central to this concept. In my initial discussion of display, I defined it as the process whereby individuals or groups of individuals 'convey to each other and to relevant others' that certain of their actions do denote family relationships.

This definition places at the heart of the concept of display the process of conveying social meanings – in this instance, meanings related to family relationships. That process is inherently interactive, and the response to actions, gestures and the use of symbols is highly relevant to our understanding of display in action. My definition makes it clear that, through processes of display individuals are conveying social meaning *to each other* as well as *to relevant others*. Thus, display is not only about conveying meaning to external agencies or seeking reactions in a public context. Indeed I give some examples in the article where it is important simply to be behaving as a family, 'doing family things', without seeking specific reactions from others. Display refers to processes which are both directly experienced by participants within the network of family relationships, and may also be observed by others outside that network.

This distinction between experiencing and observing display seems to be important in comparing the various articles in this collection. Where there are criticisms of the concept of display authors tend to be writing about the process of *observing* display, utilising examples of audiences which are external to families, including official bureaucratic audiences. They also tend to imply that examples of display must achieve a positive reaction from such audiences to be successful or valid examples of family display. If some groups or combinations of individuals find it more difficult to elicit a positive response from public audiences then, it is argued, this calls into question the value of the concept of display.

Rather than denoting an inherent flaw in the concept of display, I see this as pointing to the need for further empirical investigation. Indeed, in my original article I identified a number of questions which required further investigation including: in specific situations, whose feedback is important in reinforcing that these relationships are accepted as family-like by others not involved directly in them (Finch 2007: 75)? Chapters in this volume serve to reinforce that this remains an important area for sociological investigation.

Equally important is to re-emphasise the importance of audiences which are *within* families, rather than outside them, where display of family relationships is experienced directly rather than observed. The articles in this volume which focus attention on the 'within family' audiences tend to find the concept of display valuable and illuminating. This might suggest that the scope should be limited to internal audiences, where display is experienced directly. In my view it would be premature to conclude this without some further investigations of the more public dimensions of display, along the lines which I have discussed above.

More fundamental questions about the nature of social interactions, and the processes by which social meaning is conveyed, are also posed by this comparison between internal and external audiences. When the response of external audiences is being considered, the discussion tends to focus on the difficulties of presentation of a 'public face' of family relationships to individuals and agencies that may be deploying different frames of meaning. In these settings there is – as several authors in this collection point out – an imbalance of power in the ability to deploy or indeed to impose social meaning in the interaction. Individuals who are trying to establish that particular (in some definitions) unconventional relationships really should be seen as families can be faced with an unequal struggle, as their attempts to impose meaning of the situation are overwhelmed by broader, established cultural meanings of family relationships.

This makes sense in certain specific situations related to audiences external to families. It may well be that display is not the most appropriate concept to describe the type of social interaction which is occurring. However, when using the concept of display to analyse social interactions within families – display to internal audiences – the concept may fit more comfortably precisely because the nature of social interaction is different.

Whereas there can certainly be power imbalances within families, and actions are also interpreted by drawing on cultural frames of reference, there is also a more direct and personal basis for the interaction. In the context of interactions in families, individuals can convey meanings directly, and seek to establish or modify the shared meanings within particular family relationships. The interaction is direct, it is more intimate and crucially it takes place *over time*. The ability to establish that certain actions, gestures or forms of speech do denote affection or commitment or support does not depend on one event. Relationships have a history in which meanings are rooted, and they anticipate a future.

I welcome the variety of ways in which the articles in this volume have taken the concept of display and applied, developed and critiqued it. By refining the concept of display, questioning where it can appropriately be applied, and stimulating further empirical investigations, these articles also contribute further insights into the processes of social interaction more generally, in which participants seek to establish social meanings over time.

Bibliography

Abbot, M. W. (2001) *Problem and Non-Problem Gamblers in New Zealand: A Report on Phase Two of the 1999 National Prevalence Survey,* Wellington: Department of Internal Affairs.

Abbot, M. W. and Volberg, R. A. (2000) *Taking the Pulse on Gambling in New Zealand: Phase One of the 1999 National Prevalence Survey. Report Number Three of the New Zealand Gaming Survey,* Wellington: Department of Internal Affairs.

Abbott, M., Volberg, R., Bellringer, M. and Reith, G. (2004a) *A Review of Research on Aspects of Problem Gambling,* Prepared for the Responsibility in Gambling Trust, Gambling Research Centre, Auckland University. http://www.rigt.org.uk/downloads/Auckland_report.pdf [accessed 24 June 2005].

Abbot, M. W., Williams, M. and Volberg, R. A. (2004b) 'A Prospective Study of Problem and Non-Problem Gamblers Living in the Community', *Substance Use and Misuse,* 39, 855–84.

Adkins, L. (2002) *Revisions: Gender and Sexuality in Late Modernity,* Buckingham: Open University Press.

Alderson, P. and Morrow, V. (2004) *Ethics, Social Research and Consulting with Children and Young People,* Ilford: Barnardos.

Ali, S. (2007) 'Gendering Mixed-Race, Deconstructing Mixedness' in J. M. Sims (ed.) *Mixed Heritage – Identity, Policy and Practice,* London: Runnymede Trust.

Almack, K. (2007) 'Out and About: Negotiating the Process of Disclosure of Lesbian Parenthood', *Sociological Research Online* 12, 1. http://www. socresonline. org.uk/12/1/almack.html

Almack, K. (2008) 'Display Work: Lesbian Parent Couples and Their Families of Origin Negotiating New Kin Relationships', *Sociology,* 42, 1183–99.

Almack, K. (2011) 'Display work: Lesbian Parent Couples and Their Families of Origin Negotiating New Kin Relationships' in E. Dermott and J. Seymour (eds) *Displaying Families,* Basingstoke: Palgrave Macmillan.

Armstrong, E. (2002) *Forging Gay Identities,* Chicago, IL: Chicago University Press.

Armstrong, J. (2006) 'Beyond "Juggling" and "Flexibility": Classed and Gendered Experiences of Combining Employment and Motherhood', *Sociological Research Online*, 11, 2. http://www.socresonline.org.uk/11/2/armstrong.html

Aspinall, P., Hashem, F. and Song, M. (2008) *The Ethnic Options of 'Mixed Race' People in Britain*, ESRC End of Award Report RES-000–23–1507, Swindon: ESRC.

Austin, J. L. (1962) *How to Do Things with Words*, Oxford: Clarendon Press.

Back, L. (2007) *The Art of Listening*, Oxford and New York: Berg.

Baraitser, L. (2008) *Maternal Encounters: The Ethics of Interruption*, London: Routledge.

Barn, R. (1999) 'White Mothers, Mixed-Parentage Children and Child Welfare', *British Journal of Social Work*, 29, 269–84.

Bauman, Z. (1992) *Mortality, Immortality, and Other Life Strategies*, Stanford: Stanford University Press.

Bauman, Z. (2000) 'Shopping Around for a Place to Stay', in J. Rutherford (ed.) *The Art of Life*, London: Lawrence and Wishart.

Bauman, Z. (2003) *Liquid Love: On the Frailty of Human Bonds*, Cambridge: Polity Press.

Baxter, J. and Eyles, J. (1997) 'Evaluating Qualitative Research in Social Geography: Establishing "Rigour" in Interview Analysis', *Transactions of the Institute of British Geographers*, 22, 505–25.

Beck, U. (1992) *Risk Society: Towards a Modern Modernity*, London: Sage.

Beck, U. and Beck-Gernsheim, E. (1995) *The Normal Chaos of Love*, Cambridge: Polity Press.

Beck, U. and Beck-Gernsheim, E. (eds) (2002) *Individualization*, London: Sage.

Benmore, A. (2009) 'Behaving Appropriately: Managing Expectations of Hosts and Guests in Small Hotels in the UK' in P. A. Lynch, A. McIntosh and H. Tucker (eds) *Commercial Homes in Tourism: An International Perspective*, London: Routledge.

Bergh, C. and Kuhlhorn, E. (1994) 'Social, Psychological and Physical Consequences of Pathological Gambling in Sweden', *Journal of Gambling Studies*, 10, 275–85.

Berlant, L. (1997) 'Intimacy: A Special Issue', *Critical Inquiry*, 24, 281–8.

Bernhard, B. (2007) 'Sociological Speculations on Treating Problem Gamblers: A Clinical Sociological Imagination via a Bio-psycho-social-sociological Model', *American Behavioural Scientist*, 51, 122–38.

Berridge, V. (1990) 'The Society for the Study of Addiction 1884–1988', *British Journal of Addiction*, 85 (special issue).

Biblarz, T. J. and Stacey, J. (2010) 'How Does the Gender of Parents Matter?', *Journal of Marriage and the Family*, 72, 3–22.

Bitner, M. J. (1992) 'Servicescapes: The Impact of Physical Surroundings on Customers and Employees', *The Journal of Marketing*, 56, 57–71.

Black, D. W. and Moyer, T. (1998) 'Clinical Features and Psychiatric Comorbidity of Subjects with Pathological Gambling Behavior', *Psychiatric Services*, 49, 1434–9.

Blaszczynski, A. and McConaghy, N. (1989) 'The Medical Model of Pathological Gambling: Current Shortcomings', *Journal of Gambling Behaviour*, 5, 42–52.

Blaszczynski, A., Walker, M., Sagris, A. and Dickerson, M. (1999) 'Psychological Aspects of Gambling Behaviour: An Australian Psychological Society Position Paper', *Australian Psychologist*, 34, 4–16.

Bourdieu, P. (1977) *Outline of a Theory of Practice*, Cambridge: Cambridge University Press.

Bourdieu, P. (1984) *Distinction: A Social Critique of the Judgement of Taste*, London: Routledge.

Bourdieu, P. and Wacquant, L. (1992) *An Invitation to Reflexive Sociology*, Cambridge: Polity Press.

Bradbury, T. N. and Karney, B. R. (2010) *Intimate Relationships*, New York and London: WW Norton & Company.

Bradford, B. (2006) *Who are the 'Mixed' Ethnic Group?*, London: Office for National Statistics.

Brubaker, R., Feishchmidt, R., Fox, J. and Grancea, L. (2006) *Nationalist Politics and Everyday Ethnicity in a Transylvanian Town*, Princeton, NJ: Princeton University Press.

Butler, J. (1990) *Gender Trouble: Feminism and the Subversion of Identity*, London and New York: Routledge.

Butler, J. (1993) *Bodies that Matter*, New York: Routledge.

Byrne, B. (2006) *White Lives*, London: Routledge.

Caballero, C., Edwards, R. and Puthussery, S. (2008) *Parenting 'Mixed' Children: Negotiating Difference and Belonging in Mixed Race, Ethnicity and Faith Families*, York: Joseph Rowntree Foundation.

Carmicheal, B. A. and McClinchey, K. A. (2009) 'Exploring the Importance of Setting to the Rural Tourism Experience for Rural Commercial Home Entrepreneurs and their Guests' in P. A. Lynch, A. McIntosh and H. Tucker (eds) *Commercial Homes in Tourism. An International Perspective*, London: Routledge.

Carsten, J. (2004) *After Kinship*, Cambridge: Cambridge University Press.

Cheal, D. (2002) *Sociology of Family Life*, Basingstoke: Palgrave Macmillan.

Christensen, P., James, A. and Jenks, C. (2000) 'Home and Movement: Children constructing "Family Time"' in S. L. Holloway and G. Valentine (eds) *Children's Geographies: Playing, Living, Learning*, London: Routledge.

Ciarrocchi, J. W. and Reinert, D. F. (1993) 'Family Environment and Length of Recovery for Married Male Members of Gamblers Anonymous and Female Members of GamAnon', *Journal of Gambling Studies*, 9, 341–52.

Clarke, A. (2004) 'Maternity and Materiality: Becoming a Mother in Consumer Culture', in J. Taylor, L. Laynes and D. Wozniak (eds) *Consuming Motherhood*, New Brunswick, NJ: Rutgers University Press.

Clarke, D., Abbott, M., Tse, S., Townsend, S., Kingi, P. and Manaia, W. (2006) 'Gender, Age, Ethnic and Occupational Associations with Pathological Gambling in a New Zealand Urban Sample', *New Zealand Journal of Psychology*, 35, 84–91.

Coffey, A. and Atkinson, P. (1996) *Making Sense of Qualitative Data*, Sage: London.

Connell, R. W. (2005) *Masculinities*, Cambridge: Polity Press.

Cranny-Francis, A., Kirkby, J., Stavropoulos, P. and Waring, W. (eds) (2003) *Gender Studies: Terms and Debates*, London: Palgrave Macmillan.

Darbyshire, P., Oster, C. and Carrig, H. (2001) 'The Experience of Pervasive Loss: Children and Young People Living in a Family Where Parental Gambling Is a Problem', *Journal of Gambling Studies*, 17, 23–45.

Darke, J. and Gurney, C. (2000) 'Putting Up? Gender, Hospitality and Performance', in C. Lashley and A. Morrison (eds) *In Search of Hospitality. Theoretical Perspectives and Debates*, London: Elsevier.

D'Augelli, A. R. and Patterson, C. J. (eds) (1995) *Lesbian, Gay, and Bisexual Identities over the Lifespan: Psychological Perspectives*, Oxford: Oxford University Press.

Delphy, C. and Leonard, D. (1992) *Familiar Exploitation*, Cambridge: Polity Press.

Dennis, N. and Erdos, G. (1993) (2nd edition) *Families Without Fatherhood*, London: Institute of Economic Affairs Health and Welfare Unit.

Dermott, E. (2008) *Intimate Fatherhood*, London and New York: Routledge.

Dermott, E. and Seymour, J. (2011) 'Developing "Displaying Families": A Possibility for the Future of the Sociology of Personal Life' in E. Dermott and J. Seymour (eds) *Displaying Families*, Basingstoke: Palgrave Macmillan.

Di Domenico, M. L. and Fleming, P. (2009) '"It's a guesthouse not a brothel": Policing Sex in the Home-Workplace', *Human Relations*, 62, 245–69.

Di Domenico, M. L. and Lynch, P. (2007) 'Commercial Home Enterprises: Identity, Space and Setting' in C. Lashley, P. Lynch and A. Morrison (eds) *Hospitality: A Social Lens*, London: Elsevier.

Donovan, C., Heaphy, B. and Weeks, J. (1999) 'Citizenship and Same-Sex Relationships', *Journal of Social Policy*, 28, 689–709.

Dorrer, N., McIntosh, I., Punch, S. and Emond, R. (2010) 'Children and Food Practices in Residential Care: Ambivalence in the "Institutional" Home', *Children's Geographies*, 8, 247–59.

Dorrer, N., Punch, S., McIntosh, I. and Emond, R. (2008) 'Applying the Concept of "Display" to Food Practices and Representations of "Family" in Residential Children's Homes', BSA Family Study Group Seminar 'Displaying Families', University of Hull, 16th January.

Doucet, A. (1995) 'Gender Equality and Gender Differences in Household Work and Parenting', *Women's Studies International Forum*, 18, 271–84.

Doucet, A. (2000) 'There's a Huge Difference between Me as a Male Carer and Women: Gender, Domestic Responsibility, and the Community as an Institutional Arena', *Community Work and Family*, 3, 163–84.

Doucet, A. (2001) 'You See the Need Perhaps More Clearly Than I Have: Exploring Gendered Processes of Domestic Responsibility', *Journal of Family Issues*, 22, 328–57.

Doucet, A. (2005) '"It's Almost Like I Have a Job but I Don't Get Paid": Fathers at Home Reconfiguring Work, Care and Masculinity', *Fathering*, 2, 277–304.

Doucet, A. (2006a) *Do Men Mother?: Fatherhood, Care, and Domestic Responsibility*, Toronto: University of Toronto Press.

Doucet, A. (2006b) 'Estrogen-Filled Worlds: Fathers as Primary Caregivers and Embodiment', *Sociological Review*, 23, 695–715.

Doucet, A. (2008) '"On the Other Side of (her) Gossamer Wall": Reflexive and Relational Knowing', *Qualitative Sociology*, 31, 73–87.

Doucet, A. (2009a) 'Dad and Baby in the First Year: Gendered Embodiment', *The Annals of the American Academy of Political and Social Sciences*, 624, 78–98.

Doucet, A. (2009b) 'Gender Equality and Gender Differences: Parenting, Habitus and Embodiment', *Canadian Review of Sociology*, 48, 99–117.

Doucet, A. (2011) '"It's Just Not Good for a Man to Be Interested in Other People's Children": Fathers, Public Displays of Care, and "Relevant Others"' in E. Dermott and J. Seymour (eds) *Displaying Families*, Basingstoke: Palgrave Macmillan.

Doucet, A. (forthcoming 2012) *Bread and Roses – and the Kitchen Sink*, Toronto: University of Toronto Press.

Doucet, A., McKay, L. and Tremblay, D-G. (2009a) 'Parental Leave Policy in Canada', in S. Kamerman and P. Moss (eds) *The Politics of Parental Leave Policies: Children, Parenting, Gender and the Labour Market*, Bristol: Policy Press.

Doucet, A., McKay, L. and Tremblay, D-G. (2009b) 'Canada and Québec: Two Policies, One Country', in S. Kamerman and P. Moss (eds) *The Politics of Parental Leave Policies: Children, Parenting, Gender and the Labour Market*, Bristol: Policy Press.

Doucet, A., Tremblay, D-G. and Lero, D. (2010) 'Leave Policy and Research: Canada' in P. Moss (ed.) (revised 5th edition) *International Review of Leave Policies and Related Research*, London: Employment Relations Research.

Douglas, M. (1966) *Purity and Danger*, London: Routledge.

du Gay, P. (ed.) (1997) *The Production of Culture/Cultures of Production*, London: Sage/The Open University.

Duncan, S. and Phillips, M. (2008) 'New Families? Tradition and Change in Modern Relationships', in A. Park, J. Curtice, K. Thomson, M. Phillips, M. Johnson and E. Clery (eds) *British Social Attitudes, the 24th Report*, London: Sage.

Duncombe, J. and Marsden, D. (1993) 'Love and Intimacy: The Gender Division of Emotion and "Emotion Work"', *Sociology*, 27, 221–41.

Duncombe, J. and Marsden, D. (1999) 'Love and Intimacy: The Gender Division of Emotion and "Emotion Work"', in G. Allan (ed.) *The Sociology of Family Life*, Oxford: Blackwell.

Dunne, G. A. (2000) 'Opting into Motherhood: Lesbians Blurring the Boundaries and Transforming the Meanings of Parenthood and Kinship', *Gender and Society*, 14, 11–35.

Dunne, G. A. (2001) 'The Lady Vanishes? Reflections on the Experiences of Married and Divorced Gay Fathers', *Sociological Research Online*, 6, 1–17.

Eadington, W. R. (2004) 'The Future of Online Gambling in the United States and Elsewhere', Paper presented at the International Gambling Conference,

Gambling and Problem Gambling in New Zealand: Taking Stock and Moving Forward on Policy, Practice and Research, May, Auckland, New Zealand.

Edwards, R., Hadfield, L., Lucey, H. and Mauthner, M. (2006) *Sibling Identity and Relationships: Sisters and Brothers*, London: Routledge.

Elizur, Y. and Ziv, M. (2001) 'Family Support and Acceptance: Gay Male Identity Formation and Psychological Adjustment: A Path Model', *Family Process*, 40, 125–44.

Emmel, N. D. and Hughes, K. (2009) 'Small-N Access Cases to Refine Theories of Social Exclusion and Access to Socially Excluded Individuals and Groups' in D. Byrne and C. Ragin (eds) *The SAGE handbook of Case-Based Methods*, Sage: London.

Emmel, N., Hughes, K., and Greenhalgh, J. (2005) *Developing Methodological Strategies to Recruit and Research Socially Excluded Groups*, ESRC Research Methods Programme, November 2002–December 2005.

Emond, R. (2005) 'Ethnographic Research Methods with Children and Young People', in S. Greene and D. Hogan (eds) *Researching Children's Experiences: Approaches and Methods*, London: Sage.

Fabiansson, C. (2008) 'Pathways to Excessive Gambling – Are Young People's Approach to Gambling an Indication of Future Gambling Propensity?' *Child Indicators Research*, 1, 156–75.

Featherstone, B. (2009) *Contemporary Fathers: Theory, Policy and Practice*, Bristol: Policy Press.

Felstead, A. and Jewson, N. (2000) *In Work, at Home. Towards an Understanding of Homeworking*, London: Routledge.

Feng, Z., Boyle, P., van Ham, M. and Raab, G. (2008) 'The Neighbourhood Effect on Formation of Mixed-Ethnic Unions in Britain', paper presented at the *European Population Conference*, Barcelona, Spain, 9th–12th July.

Fiese, B. J., Foley, P. K. and Spagnola, S. (2006) 'Routines and Ritual Elements in Family Mealtimes: Contexts for Child Well-Being and Family Identity' in R.W. Larson, A.R. Wiley and K.R. Branscomb (eds) *New Directions for Child and Adolescent Development: Family Mealtime as a Context of Development and Socialization*, 111(Spring), 91–107.

Finch, J. (2007) 'Displaying Families', *Sociology*, 41, 65–81.

Finch, J. (2011) 'Afterword' in E. Dermott and J. Seymour (eds) *Displaying Families*, Basingstoke: Palgrave Macmillan.

Finch, J. and Mason, J. (1993) *Negotiating Family Responsibilities*, London: Routledge.

Finch, J. and Mason, J. (2000) *Passing on: Kinship and Inheritance in England*, London: Routledge.

Fisher, M. and Connell, R. W. M. (2002) 'Masculinities and Men in Nursing', paper presented at the *3rd College of Health Sciences Research Conference, 'From Cell to Society'*, Leura, Australia, 18th–19th September.

Fisher, S. (1993) 'Gambling and Pathological Gambling in Adolescents', *Journal of Gambling Studies*, 9, 277–88.

Fisher, S. (1999) 'A Prevalence Study of Gambling and Problem Gambling Adolescents', *Addiction Research*, 7, 509–38.

Furlong, A. and Cartmel, F. (1997) *Young People and Social Change: Individualisation and Risk in Late Modernity*, Buckingham: Open University Press.

Gabb, J. (2004a) '"I Could Eat My Baby to Bits"; Passion and Desire in Lesbian Mother-Children Love', *Gender, Place, Culture*, 11, 399–415.

Gabb, J. (2004b) 'Critical Differentials: Querying the Contrarieties between Research on Lesbian Parent Families', *Sexualities*, 7, 171–87.

Gabb, J. (2005a) 'Lesbian M/Otherhood: Strategies of Familial-Linguistic Management in Lesbian Parent Families', *Sociology*, 39, 585–603.

Gabb, J. (2005b) 'Locating Lesbian Parent Families', *Gender, Place, Culture*, 12, 419–32.

Gabb, J. (2008) *Researching Intimacy in Families*, Basingstoke: Palgrave Macmillan

Gabb, J. (2009) 'Researching Family Relationships: A Qualitative Mixed Methods Approach', *Methodological Innovations Online*, 4, 37–52.

Gabb, J. (2011) 'Troubling Displays: The Affect of Gender, Sexuality and Class', in E. Dermott and J. Seymour (eds) *Displaying Families*, Basingstoke: Palgrave Macmillan.

Gagnon, J. H. (1990) 'The Explicit and Implicit Use of the Scripting Perspective in Sex Research', *Annual Review of Sex Research*, 1, 1–43.

Gaudia, R. (1987) 'Effects of Compulsive Gambling on the Family', *Social Work*, 32, 254–6.

Getz, D., Carlsen, J. and Morrison, A. (2004) *The Family Business in Tourism and Hospitality*, London: CABI International.

Giddens, A. (1991) *Modernity and Self-identity*, Cambridge: Polity Press.

Giddens, A. (1992) *The Transformation of Intimacy: Sexuality, Love and Eroticism in Modern Societies*, Cambridge: Polity Press.

Giddens, A. (2006) 'Fate, Risk and Security' in J. F.Cosgrave (ed.) *The Sociology of Risk and Gambling Reader*, Oxford: Routledge.

Gillies, V. (2003) 'Family and Intimate Relationships: A Review of the Sociological Research', *Families and Social Capital ESRC Research Group Working Papers*, No. 2.

Gillies, V. (2006) *Marginalised Mothers. Exploring Working Class Experiences of Parenting*, London: Routledge.

Gillies, V., Ribbens-McCarthy, J. and Holland, J. (2001) *Pulling Together, Pulling Apart: the Family Lives of Young People*, London: Family Policy Centre/JRF.

Gillis, J. (1996) *A World of Their Own Making. Myth, Ritual, and the Quest for Family Values*, Cambridge: Harvard University Press.

Gittins, D. (1993) *The Family in Question*, London: Macmillan.

Griffiths, M. (2001) 'Internet Gambling: Preliminary Results of the first U.K. Prevalence Study' *E-Gambling: The Electronic Journal of Gambling Issues*, 5. http://www.camh.net/egambling/issue5/research/griffiths_article.html

Griffiths, M. and Parke, J. (2002) 'The Social Impact of Internet Gambling', *Social Science Computer Review*, 20, 312–20.

Gross, N. (2005) 'The Detraditionalization of Intimacy Reconsidered', *Sociological Theory* 23, 286–311.

Gurney, C. (1999) '"We've Got Friends Who Live in Council Houses": Power and Resistance in Home Ownership', in J. Hearn and S. Roseneil (eds) *Consuming Cultures: Power and Resistance*, London: Macmillan.

Haldar, M. and Waerdahl, R. (2009) 'Teddy Diaries: A Method for Studying the Display of Family Life', *Sociology*, 43, 1141–50.

Haldrup, M. and Larsen, J. (2003) 'The Family Gaze', *Tourist Studies*, 3, 32–46.

Hall, C.M. (2009) 'Sharing Space with Visitors: The Servicescape of the Commercial Exurban Home' in P. A. Lynch, A. McIntosh and H. Tucker (eds) *Commercial Homes in Tourism. An International Perspective*, London: Routledge.

Hall, S. (1980) 'Encoding/Decoding', in S. Hall, D. Hobson, A. Lowe and P. Willis (eds) *Culture, Media, Language, Working Papers in Cultural Studies 1972–79*, London: Hutchinson.

Hansen, K. V. (2005) *Not-So-Nuclear Families: Class, Gender and Networks of Care*, Piscataway, NJ: Rutgers University Press.

Hardyment, C. (2007) *Dream Babies: Childcare Advice from John Locke to Gina Ford*, London: Francis Lincoln.

Haynes, J. and Dermott, E. (2011) 'Displaying Mixedness: Difference and Family Relationships' in E. Dermott and J. Seymour (eds) *Displaying Families*, Basingstoke: Palgrave Macmillan.

Haynes J., Tikly, L. and Caballero, C. (2006) 'The Barriers to Achievement for White/Black Caribbean Pupils in English Schools', *British Journal of Sociology of Education*, 27, 569–83.

Heaphy, B. (2007) *Late Modernity and Social Change: Reconstructing Social and Personal Life*. London: Routledge.

Heaphy, B. (2011) 'Critical Relational Displays', in E. Dermott and J. Seymour (eds) *Displaying Families*, Basingstoke: Palgrave Macmillan.

Heaphy, B. and Yip, A. (2006) 'Policy Implications of Ageing Sexualities', *Social Policy and Society*, 5, 1–9.

Held, V. (1993) *Feminist Morality: Transforming Culture, Society and Politics*, Chicago, IL: University of Chicago Press.

Held, V. (2005) *The Ethics of Care: Personal, Political and Global*, Oxford: Oxford University Press.

Holloway, S. and Valentine, G. (2002) *Cyberkids: Children in the Information Age*, London: Routledge.

Hughes, K. (2007) 'Migrating Identities: The Relational Constitution of Drug Use and Addiction', *Sociology of Health and Illness*, 29, 1–19.

Hughes, K. and Valentine, G. (2011) 'Practices of Display: the Framing and Changing of Internet Gambling Behaviours in Families', in E. Dermott and J. Seymour (eds) *Displaying Families*, Basingstoke: Palgrave Macmillan.

Ingraham, C. (1996) 'The Heterosexual Imaginary. Feminist Sociology and Theories of Gender' in S. Seidman (ed.) *Queer Theory/Sociology*, Oxford: Blackwell.

Irwin, S. (2005) *Reshaping Social Life*, London and New York: Routledge.

Jackson, P. (2009) 'Introduction: Food as a Lens on Family Life' in P. Jackson (ed.) *Changing Families, Changing Food*, Houndmills: Palgrave Macmillan.

James, A. (2007) 'A Proper Dinner', *Times Higher Education Supplement*, 25th May.

James, A. and Curtis, P. (2010) 'Family Displays and Personal Lives', *Sociology*, 44, 1163–80.

Jamieson, L. (1998) *Intimacy: Personal Relationships in Modern Societies*, Cambridge: Polity Press.

Jamieson, L. (2005) 'Intimacy' in Ritzer, G. (ed.) *Encyclopedia of Sociology*, Oxford: Blackwell.

Jenkins, R. (1994) 'Rethinking Ethnicity: Identity, Categorization and Power', *Ethnic and Racial Studies*, 17, 197–223.

Jennings, G. (2009) 'All at Sea: When the Commercial Home is a Sailing Boat', in P. A. Lynch, A. McIntosh and H. Tucker (eds) *Commercial Homes in Tourism. An International Perspective*, London: Routledge.

Johnston, L. and Valentine, G. (1995) 'Wherever I Lay My Girlfriend, That's My Home' in D. Bell and G. Valentine (eds) *Mapping Desire: Geographies of Sexualities*, London: Routledge.

Jovchelovitch, S. (2006) *Knowledge in Context: Representations, Community and Culture*, London: Routledge.

Kalischuk, R. G., Nowatzki, N., Cardwell, K., Klein, K. and Solowoniuk, J. (2006) 'Problem Gambling and Its Impact on Families: A Literature Review', *International Gambling Studies*, 6, 31–60.

Kehily, M-J. and Thomson, R. (2011) 'Displaying Motherhood: Representations, Visual Methods and the Materiality of Maternal Practice' in E. Dermott and J. Seymour (eds) *Displaying Families*, Basingstoke: Palgrave Macmillan.

Klesse, C. (2007) *The Spectre of Promiscuity*, London: Ashgate.

Knapp Whittier, D. K. and Melendez, R. M. (2004) 'Intersubjectivity in the Intrapsychic Sexual Scripting of Gay Men', *Culture, Health and Sexuality*, 6, 131–43.

Krishnan, M. and Orford, J. (2002) 'Gambling and the Family: From the Stress-Coping-Support Perspective', *International Gambling Studies*, 2, 61–83.

Larson, R. W., Branscomb, K. R. and Wiley, A. R. (2006) 'Forms and Functions of Family Mealtimes: Multidisciplinary Perspectives' in R.W. Larson, A. R. Wiley and K. R. Branscomb (eds) *New Directions for Child and Adolescent Development: Family Mealtime as a Context of Development and Socialization*, 111(Spring), 91–107.

Lashley, C., Lynch, P. and Morrison, A. (eds) (2007) *Hospitality: A Social Lens*, London: Elsevier.

Law, J. (2004) *After Method: Mess in Social Science Research*, London: Routledge.

Lesieur, H. R. (1984). *The Chase: Career of the Compulsive Gambler*. Cambridge, MA: Schenkman Publishing Co.

Lesieur, H. and Rosenthal, R. (1991) 'Pathological Gambling: A Review of the Literature', *Journal of Gambling Studies*, 7, 5–39.

Lindsay, J., Perlesz, A., Brown, R., McNair, R., de Vaus, D. and Pitts, M. (2006), 'Stigma or Respect: Lesbian-Parented Families Negotiating School Settings', *Sociology*, 40, 1059–77.

Longmore, M. A. (1998) 'Symbolic Interactionism and the Study of Sexuality', *Journal of Sex Research*, 35, 45–57.

Lorenz, V. C. and Yaffee, R. A (1988) 'Pathological Gambling: Psychosomatic, Emotional and Marital Difficulties as reported by the Spouse', *Journal of Gambling Behaviour*, 4, 13–26.

Luxton, M. (1980/2010) *More than a Labour of Love: Three Generations of Women's Work in the Home*, Toronto, Canada: Women's Educational Press.

Luxton, M. and Vosko, L. F. (1998) 'The Census and Women's Work', *Studies in Political Economy*, 56, 49–82.

Lynch, M. (2000) 'Against Reflexivity as an Academic Virtue and Source of Privileged Knowledge', *Theory, Culture and Society*, 17, 26–54.

Lynch, P. A. (2005) 'The Commercial Home Enterprise and Host: A United Kingdom Perspective', *International Journal of Hospitality Management*, 24, 533–53.

Lynch, P. A., McIntosh, A. and Tucker, H. (eds) (2009a) *Commercial Homes in Tourism. An International Perspective*, London: Routledge.

Lynch, P. A., McIntosh, A. and Tucker, H. (2009b) 'Introduction' in Lynch, P.A., McIntosh, A. and Tucker, H. (eds) *Commercial Homes in Tourism. An International Perspective*, London: Routledge.

Lynch, P. A., McIntosh, A. and Tucker, H. (2009c) 'Conclusions and Research Considerations' in Lynch, P. A., McIntosh, A. and Tucker, H. (eds) *Commercial Homes in Tourism. An International Perspective*, London: Routledge.

Marshall, K. (2009) 'The Family Work Week', *Perspectives on Labour and Income (Statistics Canada catalogue no. 75–001-XPE)*, 21(Summer), 21–9.

Martens, L. (2009) 'Creating the Ethical Parent-Consumer Subject: Commerce, Moralities and Pedagogies in Early Parenthood' in J. A. Sandlin and P. McLaren (eds) *Critical Pedagogies of Consumption: Living and Learning in the Shadow of the "Shopocalypse"*, New York: Routledge.

Mason, J. (2004) 'Personal Narratives, Relational Selves: Residential Histories in the Living and Telling', *The Sociological Review*, 52, 162–79.

Mason, J. (2008) 'Tangible Affinities and the Real Life Fascination of Kinship', *Sociology*, 42, 29–45.

Mauthner, N. S. and Doucet, A. (2003) 'Reflexive Accounts and Accounts of Reflexivity in Qualitative Data Analysis', *Sociology*, 37, 413–31.

May, C. (2001) 'Pathology, Identity and the Social Construction of Alcohol Dependence', *Sociology*, 33, 2, 385–401.

McIntosh, I., Dorrer, N., Emond, R. and Punch, S. (2010) '"You Don't Have to be Watched to Make Your Toast": Surveillance and Food Practices within Residential Care', *Surveillance and Society*, 7, 290–303.

McIntosh, I., Dorrer, N., Punch, S. and Emond, R. (2011) '"I Know We Can't Be a Family, but as Close as You Can Get": Displaying Families within an Institutional Context' in E. Dermott and J. Seymour (eds) *Displaying Families*, Basingstoke: Palgrave Macmillan.

McIntosh, J. and McKeganey, N. (2000) 'Addicts' Narratives of Recovery from Drug Use: Constructing a Non-Addict Identity', *Social Science and Medicine*, 50, 1501–10.

216 *Bibliography*

McKay, L. and Doucet, A. (2010) '"Without Taking Away Her Leave": A Canadian Case Study of Couples' Decisions on Fathers' Use of Paid Leave', *Fathering*, 10, 300–20.

McKay, L., Marshall, K. and Doucet, A. (2011) 'Fathers and Parental Leave in Canada: Policies, Practices and Potential' in J. Ball and K. Daly (eds) *Engaging Fathers in Social Change: Lessons from Canada*, Vancouver: UBC Press.

McKie, L., Cunningham-Burley, S. and McKendrick, J. (2005) 'Families and Relationships: Boundaries and Bridges', in L. McKie and S. Cunningham-Burley (eds) *Families in Society: Boundaries and Relationships*, Bristol: The Policy Press.

McLeod, J. and Thomson, R. (2009) *Researching Social Change: Qualitative Approaches*, London: Sage.

McPheat, G., Milligan, I. and Hunter, L. (2007) 'What's the Use of Residential Childcare? Findings of Two Studies Detailing Current Trends in the Use of Residential Childcare in Scotland', *Journal of Children's Services*, 2, 15–25.

Merin, Y. (2002) *Equality for Same Sex Couples: The Legal Recognition of Gay Partnerships in Europe and the United States*, Chicago, IL: University of Chicago Press.

Mingione, E. (1988) 'Work and Informal Activities in Urban Southern Italy' in R. E. Pahl (ed.) *On Work: Historical, Comparative and Theoretical Approaches*, Oxford: Basil Blackwell.

Morgan, D. H. J. (1996) *Family Connections: An Introduction to Family Studies*, Cambridge: Polity Press.

Morgan, D. H. J. (1999) 'Risk and Family Practices: Accounting for Change and Fluidity in Family Life' in E. B. Silva and C. Smart (eds) *The New Family?*, London: Sage Publications.

Morgan, D. H. J. (2009) *Acquaintances: The Space between Intimates and Strangers*, Maidenhead: Open University Press.

Moscovici, S. (2000) *Social Representations: Studies in Social Psychology*, Cambridge: Polity Press.

Murray, C. (1990) *The Emerging British Underclass*, London: Institute for Economic Affairs.

Murray, C. (1996) *Charles Murray and the Underclass: The Developing Debate*, London: Institute for Economic Affairs.

Nayak, A. (2006) 'Displaced Masculinities: Chavs, Youth and Class in the Post Industrial City', *Sociology*, 40, 813–31.

Ochs, E. and Shohet, M. (2006) 'The Cultural Structuring of Mealtime Socialization' in R. W. Larson, A. R. Wiley and K. R. Branscomb (eds) *New Directions for Child and Adolescent Development: Family Mealtime as a Context of Development and Socialization*, 111 (Spring), 35–49.

Okin, S. M. (1989) *Justice, Gender and the Family*, New York: Basic Books.

Orford, J. (1994) 'Empowering Family and Friends: A New Approach to the Secondary Prevention of Addiction', *Drug & Alcohol Review*, 13, 417–29.

Owen, C. (2007) 'Statistics: The Mixed Category in Census 2001' in J. M. Sims (ed.) *Mixed Heritage – Identity, Policy and Practice*, London: Runnymede Trust.

Pahl, R. E. (1984) *Divisions of Labour*, Oxford: Basil Blackwell.

Penelope, J. and Wolfe, S. (1989) *The Original Coming Out Stories*, Freedom, CA: Crossing Press.

Perusse, D. (2003) 'New Maternity and Parental Benefits', *Perspectives on Labour and Income (Statistics Canada catalogue no. 75–001-XIE)*, 4, 1–4.

Petry, N. M. (2006) 'Internet Gambling: An Emerging Concern in Family Practice Medicine?', *Family Practice*, 23, 421–6.

Phillips, M. (1998) 'The Truth That Dare Not Speak Its Name', *The Observer*, 27th February.

Platt, L. (2009) *Ethnicity and Family: Relationships within and between Ethnic Groups: An Analysis using the Labour Force Survey*, London: Equality and Human Rights Commission.

Plummer, K. (ed.) (1992) *Modern Homosexualities: Fragments of Lesbian and Gay Experience*, London: Routledge.

Plummer, K. (1995) *Telling Sexual Stories: Power, Change and Social Worlds*, London: Routledge.

Plummer, K. (2003) *Intimate Citizenship: Private Decisions and Public Dialogues*, Seattle WA and London: University of Washington Press.

Presser, L. (2004) 'Violent Offenders, Moral Selves: Constructing Identities and Accounts in the Research Interview', *Social Problems*, 51, 82–101.

Punch, S. (2002) 'Research with Children: The Same or Different from Research with Adults?', *Childhood*, 9, 321–41.

Punch, S., McIntosh, I. and Emond, R. (2010) 'Children's Food Practices in Families and Institutions', *Children's Geographies*, 8, 227–32.

Punch, S., McIntosh, I., Emond, R. and Dorrer, N. (2009) 'Food and Relationships: Children's Experiences in Residential Care', in A. James, A. T. Kjørholt and V. Tingstad (eds) *Children, Food and Identity in Everyday Life*, Basingstoke: Palgrave Macmillan.

Quinn, F. L. (2001) 'First Do no Harm: What Could Be Done by Casinos to Limit Pathological Gambling', *Managerial and Decision Economics*, 22, 133–42.

Ramazanoglu, C. and Holland, J. (2002) *Feminist Methodology*, London: Sage.

Ranson, G. (2010) *Against the Grain: Couples, Gender and the Reframing of Parenting*, Toronto: University of Toronto Press.

Reith, G. (1999) *The Age of Chance: Gambling in Western Culture*, Routledge: London.

Ribbens McCarthy, J. and Edwards, R. (2002) 'The Individual in the Public and Private: the Significance of Mothers and Children', in A. Carling, S. Duncan and R. Edwards (eds) *Analysing Families: Morality and Rationality in Policy and Practice*, London: Routledge.

Ribbens McCarthy, J., Edwards, R. and Gillies, V. (2003) *Making Families: Moral Tales of Parenting and Step-Parenting*, York: Sociology Press.

Roseneil, S. (2007) 'Queer Individualization: The Transformation of Personal Life in the Early 21st Century', *Nora, Nordic Journal of Women's Studies*, 15, 84–99.

Ruddick, S. (1995) *Maternal Thinking: Towards a Politics of Peace*, Boston, MA: Beacon Press.

Ryan-Flood, R. (2005) 'Contested Heteronormativities: Discourses of Fatherhood among Lesbian Parents in Sweden and Ireland', *Sexualities*, 8, 189–204.

Ryan-Flood, R. (2009) *Lesbian Motherhood: Gender, Families and Sexual Citizenship*, Basingstoke: Palgrave Macmillan.

Ryan-Flood, R. (2011) 'Commentary on Almack's Chapter' in E. Dermott and J. Seymour (eds) *Displaying Families*, Basingstoke: Palgrave Macmillan.

Sargent, P. (2000) 'Real Men or Real Teachers? Contradictions in the Lives of Men Elementary Teachers', *Men and Masculinities*, 2, 410–33.

Selwyn, J., Harris, P., Quinton, D., Nawaz, S., Wijedasa, D. and Wood, M. (2008) *Pathways to Permanence for Black, Asian and Mixed Ethnicity Children: Dilemmas, Decision-making and Outcomes*, London: Department for Children, Schools and Families.

Selwyn, T. (2000) 'An Anthropology of Hospitality', in Lashley, C. and Morrison, A. (eds) *In Search of Hospitality. Theoretical Perspectives and Debates*, London: Elsevier.

Seymour, J. (2005) 'Entertaining Guests or Entertaining the Guests: Children's Emotional Labour in Hotels, Pubs and Boarding Houses', in J. Goddard, S. McNamee, A. L. James and A. James (eds) *The Politics of Childhood. International Perspectives, Contemporary Developments*, London: Palgrave Macmillan.

Seymour, J. (2007) 'Treating the Hotel like a Home: The Contribution of Studying the Single Location Home/workplace', *Sociology*, 41, 1097–114.

Seymour, J. (2011) '"Family Hold Back": Displaying Families in the Single Location Home/Workplace' in E. Dermott and J. Seymour (eds) *Displaying Families*, Basingstoke: Palgrave Macmillan.

Seymour, J. (forthcoming) *Family Practices and Spatiality*, Basingstoke: Palgrave Macmillan.

Shaffer, H. J. (1999) 'Strange Bedfellows: A Critical View of Pathological Gambling and Addiction', *Addiction*, 94, 1445–8.

Short, L. (2007a) 'Lesbian Mothers Living Well in the Context of Heterosexism and Discrimination: Resources, Strategies and Legislative Change', *Feminism & Psychology*, 17, 57–74.

Short, L. (2007b) '"It Makes the World of Difference": Benefits for Children of Lesbian Parents of Having their Parents Legally Recognised as their Parents', *Gay & Lesbian Issues and Psychology Review*, 3, 5–15.

Short, L. (2011) 'Commentary on Almack' in E. Dermott and J. Seymour (eds) *Displaying Families*, Basingstoke: Palgrave Macmillan.

Silva, E. B. and Smart, C. (eds) (1999) *The New Family*, London: Sage.

Silva, E. B. and Smart, C. (1999) 'The "New" Practices and Politics of Family Life', in E. B. Silva and C. Smart (eds) *The New Family*, London: Sage.

Simon, W. and Gagnon, J. H. (1986) 'Sexual Scripts: Permanence and Change', *Archives of Sexual Behavior*, 15 (2), 97–120.

Simon, W. and Gagnon, J. H. (2003) 'Sexual Scripts: Origins, Influences and Changes', *Qualitative Sociology*, 26 (4), 491–7.

Sims, J. M. (ed.) (2007) *Mixed Heritage: Identity, Policy and Practice*, London: Runnymede Trust.

Skeggs, B. (2004) *Class, Self, Culture*, London: Routledge.

Sloane-White, P. (2009) 'The Hospitable Muslim Home in Urban Malaysia: A Sociable Site for Economic and Political Action' in P. A. Lynch, A. McIntosh and H. Tucker (eds) *Commercial Homes in Tourism. An International Perspective*, London: Routledge.

Smart, C. (2007) *Personal Life: New Directions in Sociological Thinking*, Cambridge: Polity Press.

Smart, C. and Neale, B. (1999) *Family Fragments?*, Cambridge: Polity Press.

Smart, C. and Shipman, B. (2004) 'Vision in Monochrome: Families, Marriage and the Individualization Thesis', *British Journal of Sociology*, 55, 491–509.

Smith, A. M. (1997) 'The Good Homosexual and the Dangerous Queer: Resisting the "New Homophobia"' in L. Segal (ed.) *New Sexual Agendas*, London: Palgrave Macmillan.

Smith, J. A. (2009) *The Daddy Shift: How Stay-at-Home Dads, Breadwinning Moms, and Shared Parenting Are Transforming the American Family*, Boston, MA: Beacon Press.

Smith, M. (2009) *Rethinking Residential Child Care: Positive Perspectives*, Bristol: Policy Press.

Song, M. (2003) *Choosing Ethnic Identity*, Cambridge: Blackwell.

Song, M. (2007) 'The Diversity of "the" Mixed Race Population in Britain', Mixedness and Mixing: New Perspectives on Mixed-Race Britons, Commission for Racial Equality Conference, 4th–6th September. http://mixedness.millipedia.net/Default.aspx.LocID-0hgnew0yr.RefLocID-0hg01l0hg01l001.Lang-EN.htm

Southerton, D. (2009) *Communities of Consumption*, Saarbrücken, Germany: VDM Verlag.

Stacey, J. (1990) *Brave New Families: Stories of Domestic Upheaval in Late Twentieth Century America*, New York: Basic Books.

Stacey, J. and Biblarz, T. J. (2001) '(How) Does The Sexual Orientation of Parents Matter?', *American Sociological Review*, 66, 159–83.

Statistics Canada (2002) *Annual Average 2002 Family Characteristics of Single Husband-Wife Families, Labour Force Survey*, Ottawa: Statistics Canada.

Statistics Canada (2009) *Labour Force Survey*, Unpublished data.

Steel, Z. and Blaszczynski, A. (1998) 'Impulsivity, Personality Disorders and Pathological Gambling Severity', *Addiction*, 93, 895–905.

Steier, F. (ed.) (1991) *Research and Reflexivity*, London: Sage.

Stonequist, E. V. (1937) *The Marginal Man: A Study of Personality and Culture Conflict*, New York: Russell and Russell.

Sussman, D. and Bonnell, S. (2006) 'Wives as Primary Breadwinners', *Statistics Canada: Perspectives on Labour and Income*, 7.

Taylor, Y. (2009) *Lesbian and Gay Parenting: Securing Social and Educational Capital*, London: Palgrave Macmillan.

Thomson, R. and Kehily, M. J. (2009) 'The Making of Modern Motherhoods: Storying an Emergent Identity' in M. Wetherell (ed.) *Liveable Lives: Negotiating Identities in New Times*, Basingstoke: Palgrave Macmillan.

Thorne, B. (1993) *Gender Play: Girls and Boys in School*, Buckingham: Open University Press.

Tikly, L., Caballero, C., Haynes, J. and Hill, J. (2004) *Understanding the Educational Needs of Mixed Heritage Pupils*, London: Department for Education and Skills.

Tyler, I. (2001) 'Skin-tight: Celebrity, Pregnancy and Subjectivity' in S. Ahmed and J. Stacey (eds) *Thinking Through the Skin*, London: Routledge.

Tyler, I. (2008) 'Chav Mum, Chav Scum: Class Disgust in Contemporary Britain', *Feminist Media Studies*, 8, 17–34.

Valentine, G. and Hughes, K. (2008) *New Forms of Participation: Problem Internet Gambling and the Role of the Family.* http://www.lssi.leeds.ac.uk/getfile.php?file=pdf_26

Valentine, G. and Hughes, K. (2010) 'Ripples in a Pond: The Disclosure to, and Management of, Problem Internet Gambling with/in the Family', *Community, Work & Family*, 1469–3615, 13 (3), 273–90.

Valentine, G., Skelton, T. and Butler, R. (2003) 'Coming Out and Outcomes: Negotiating Lesbian and Gay Identities with, and in, the Family', *Environment and Planning D: Society and Space*, 21, 479–99.

Van Every, J. (1999) 'From Modern Nuclear Family Households to Postmodern Diversity? The Sociological Construction of "Families"' in G. Jagger and C. Wright (eds) *Changing Family Values*, London: Routledge.

Volberg, R. A. (1994) 'The Prevalence and Demographics of Pathological Gamblers: Implications for Public Health', *American Journal of Public Health*, 84, 237–41.

Volberg, R. A. (2000) 'The Future of Gambling in the United Kingdom: Increasing Access Creates more Problem Gamblers', *British Medical Journal*, 320, 7249.

Wallace, C. D. and Pahl, R. E. (1985) 'Household Work Strategies in an Economic Recession' in N. Redclift and E. Mingione (eds) *Beyond Employment*, Oxford: Basil Blackwell.

Ward, J. (2004) '"Not all Differences Are Created Equal": Multiple Jeopardy in a Gendered Organization', *Gender and Society*, 18 (1), 82–102.

Wardle, H., Sproston, K., Orford, J., Erens, B., Griffiths, M., Constantine, R. and Pigott, S. (2007) *The British Gambling Prevalence Survey*, Birmingham: The Gambling Commission. www.gamblingcommission.gov.uk

Weeks, J. (1991) *Against Nature*, London: Rivers Oram.

Weeks, J., Heaphy, B. and Donovan, C. (2001) *Same Sex Intimacies: Families of Choice and Other Life Experiments*, London: Routledge.

Welte, J., Barnes, G., Wieczorek, W., Tidwell, M. and Parker, J. (2001) 'Alcohol and Gambling Pathology among U.S Adults: Prevalence, Demographic Patterns and Comorbidity', *Journal of Studies on Alcohol*, 62, 706–12.

Weston, K. (1991 and 1997, revised version) *Families We Choose: Lesbians, Gays, Kinship*, New York: Columbia University Press.

Williams, C. L. (1992) 'The Glass Escalator: Hidden Advantage for Men in the "Female" Professions', *Social Problems*, 39, 253–67.

Williams, F. (2004) *Rethinking Families*, London: Calouste Gulbenkian Foundation.

Willis, P., Jones, S., Canaan, J. and Hurd, G. (1990) *Common Culture: Symbolic Work at Play in the Everyday Cultures of the Young*, Maidenhead: Open University Press.

Wood, R. T. A. and Griffiths, M. D. (2007) 'Time Loss whilst Playing Video Games: Is There a Relationship to Addictive Behaviours?', *International Journal of Mental Health and Addiction*, 5, 141–9.

Yellowlees, P. M. and Marks, S. (2005) 'Problematic Internet Use or Internet Addiction', *Computers in Human Behaviour*, 23, 1447–53.

Yip, A. K. T. (2004) 'Negotiating Space within Family and Kin in Identity Construction: The Narratives of British Non-heterosexual Muslims', *Sociological Review*, 52, 336–49.

Young, I. M. (1990) *Justice and the Politics of Difference*, Princeton, NJ: PrincetonUniversity Press.

Young, I. M. (1997) *Intersecting Voices: Dilemmas of Gender, Political Philosophy, and Policy*, Princeton, NJ: Princeton University Press.

Young, I. M. (2005) 'House and Home: Feminist Variations on a Theme' in S. Hardy and C. Wiedmer (eds) *Motherhood and Space: Configurations of the Maternal Through Politics, Home and the Body*, Basingstoke: Palgrave Macmillan.

Author Index

Subject Index